T0355902

KISS YOUR DENTIST GOODBYE

A DO-IT-YOURSELF MOUTH CARE SYSTEM FOR HEALTHY, CLEAN GUMS AND TEETH

SECOND EDITION

ELLIE PHILLIPS, DDS

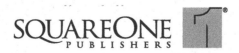

SQUAREONE
PUBLISHERS

The information and advice contained in this book are based upon the research and the personal and professional experiences of the author. They are not intended as a substitute for consulting with a healthcare professional. The publisher and author are not responsible for any adverse effects or consequences resulting from the use of any of the suggestions, preparations, or procedures discussed in this book. All matters pertaining to your physical health should be supervised by a healthcare professional. It is a sign of wisdom, not cowardice, to seek a second or third opinion.

EDITOR: Anthony Pomes • TYPESETTER: Gary A. Rosenberg

Square One Publishers
115 Herricks Road • Garden City Park, NY 11040
(516) 535-2010 • (877) 900-BOOK • www.squareonepublishers.com

Library of Congress Cataloging-in-Publication Data
Names: Phillips, Ellie, author.
Title: Kiss your dentist goodbye : healthy, clean gums and teeth / Ellie, DDS
    Phillips.
Description: Second edition. | Garden City Park : Square One Publishers, 2025.
    | Includes bibliographical references and index. | Summary: "In this book,
    Dr. Phillips emphasizes explains the importance of bacterial balance for oral
    health, highlighting how it will never be attained through excessive flossing,
    aggressive cleanings, or the indiscriminate killing of mouth bacteria. She
    exposes the detrimental effects of certain dental procedures and products,
    including tooth whitening, bleaching, dental sealants, and certain fluorides. By
    adopting her practical do-it-yourself daily routine, you can effortlessly reduce
    plaque buildup, strengthen your teeth, heal and even reverse small cavities, cure
    periodontal disease, and eliminate tooth sensitivity"— Provided by publisher.
Identifiers: LCCN 2024047734 | ISBN 9780757005312 (paperback) | ISBN
    9780757055317 (epub)
Subjects: LCSH: Teeth—Care and hygiene.
Classification: LCC RK61 .P535 2025 | DDC 617.6—dc23/eng/20241120
LC record available at https://lccn.loc.gov/2024047734

Copyright © 2025 by Ellie Phillips

All rights reserved. No part of this publication may be reproduced, stored in a retrieval system, or transmitted, in any form or by any means, electronic, mechanical, photocopying, recording, or otherwise, without the prior written permission of the publisher. Furthermore, no existing portions of the copyrighted material contain herein shall be repurposed or drawn upon by any/all present or future forms of AI (artificial intelligence) systems/applications worldwide.

Printed in the United States of America

10   9   8   7   6   5   4   3   2   1

"Truly Life-Changing"

"I vividly remember picking up the first edition of this book and reading it cover to cover in one sitting—it was incredible and truly life-changing. As a pediatric dentist, I frequently explain to parents that baby teeth are critical to the proper development of adult oral health. Dental disease is entirely preventable, and it's vital for parents to understand that unnecessary or invasive treatments in a child's mouth can have long-term consequences on their oral health. I would love to see dental education place greater emphasis on the types of effective, non-invasive, and preventative strategies detailed in this outstanding book."

DR. QUINN YOST, DDS, MSD • BOARD-CERTIFIED PEDIATRIC DENTIST

"For Anyone Seeking to Improve Their Dental Health"

"Your mouth is the first place where your food gets its chance to help or harm your health—starting with your teeth and gums! In this second edition of *Kiss Your Dentist Goodbye*, Dr. Phillips gives valuable advice that everyone needs to know on how to optimize their oral health. She has your back, so read this book to kiss *your fear* of the dentist goodbye."

DR. WILLIAM W. LI, MD • *NEW YORK TIMES* BESTSELLING AUTHOR OF *EAT TO BEAT DISEASE* AND *EAT TO BEAT YOUR DIET*, AND PRESIDENT AND MEDICAL DIRECTOR, THE ANGIOGENESIS FOUNDATION

"A Clear and Lucid Guide"

"Dr. Ellie's passion for healthier teeth is limitless, and this book clearly explains the impact of an unhealthy mouth on body health. My passion for prevention includes women's heart health, and Dr. Ellie explains why women's teeth suffer in a special way as they are affected by dramatic shifts in mouth pH and dryness over time. This informative new second edition of *Kiss Your Dentist Goodbye* is a clear and lucid guide filled with all kinds of action-based tips and protocols. Thank you, Dr. Ellie."

DR. AMY DONEEN, DNP, ARNP • MEDICAL DIRECTOR, THE PREVENTION CENTER FOR HEART & BRAIN HEALTH

"For Patients to Be Empowered"

"I interviewed Dr. Phillips as part of a story for *The Times* (of London) covering flossing. Her evidence-based debunking of the myths around flossing went completely against decades of public health education, but Dr. Phillips was right. The research was incontrovertible, and backed up by my own adoption of her methods. I also became acutely aware, as this book describes, of a disconnect in the world of patient education, and the need for patients to be empowered about their oral health and effective strategies to use at home, between dental visits.

HELEN RUMBELOW, JOURNALIST, *THE TIMES* OF LONDON, UK

"So Much for Consumers to Learn"

"The message in this book is about the impact of poor oral health on oral and general health, but it also addresses the dangerous oral health spiral that can begin with just a few small fillings. There is so much for consumers to learn—and easy behavior changes that everyone can use to achieve oral health success. This book offers an in-depth picture of the pivotal role xylitol plays in the prevention of dental disease. It is of particular value for expectant parents if they read it *before* their baby is born."

TRISHA E. O'HEHIR, MS, RDH, PRESIDENT OF O'HEHIR UNIVERSITY, BUTEYKO BREATHING COACH

"Impressive"

"This book challenges us to consider the impact of plastics, metals, and oral diseases on overall health. It advocates for a shift in how we approach oral care, with deeper evaluations and higher expectations for what dentistry should be in America. Dr. Ellie Phillips' impressive work is bound to start meaningful conversations we should have started long ago."

DR. HOWARD FARRAN, DDS, MBA, PUBLISHER, FOUNDER OF DENTALTOWN, HOST OF *DENTISTRY UNCENSORED* PODCAST

"I Love This Book"

"I love this book! Dr. Ellie has tackled a difficult subject—the simplification of oral health—and has done the job well. As a dentist, there is much to learn, and this new edition of her vital and invaluable book adds many new dimensions to the topic of oral health, making it a book for all patients—and even your dentist—to enjoy."

DR. JOHN FOCHELLA, DMD, DENTAL SPECIALIST AND LECTURER

"Invaluable"

"This invaluable resource is a must-read for anyone looking to better understand their dental health journey. Dr. Ellie skillfully breaks down the key information patients need to know—not just about what a dental visit entails, but about the empowering choices they have when it comes to their care. Her insights into when to delay or refuse treatments, and how to address the myriad of microbes in the mouth, are both enlightening and practical. I'm confident that dental professionals and their patients alike will find this book to be an essential guide in navigating the modern dental landscape. It's a perfect recommendation for those seeking to take control of their oral health in a more informed, personalized way!"

DIANE LARSON, RDH, BSDH, DIRECTOR OF
CLINICAL EDUCATION AT ORALDNA LABS

"Will Shine a Light on These New Treatment Options"

"Dr. Ellie always says it like it is—and here she is again, speaking uncomfortable truths in this brand new edition of *Kiss Your Dentist Goodbye*. In this book, Dr. Ellie has informed patients about these possibilities for change and the techniques dentists can implement for 'no-drill, no-fear' dentistry in their offices. I know this book will shine a light on these new treatment options that give patients what *they* want."

DR. CHRIS KAMMER, DDS, FOUNDER OF THE AMERICAN
ACADEMY FOR ORAL SYSTEMIC HEALTH

"Here Are So Many Ways People Can Help Themselves"

"In this book, Dr. Ellie Phillips has built a bridge across the chasm of oral health self-care knowledge that has unfortunately existed between dental science and the public. People are suffering and dentistry needs to do better. As a leader in the use of medicines to treat and prevent cavities worldwide, I spent a decade searching for drugs to stop cavities but found the answer in nutrients from foods. People deserve to know that cavities and gum disease are diseases, like other medical diseases, and they can be halted with effective strategies. Here are so many ways people can help themselves, and ways for dentists to make treatments less invasive, easier, and more comfortable."

JEREMY HORST KEEPER, DDS, MS, PHD
PAST DIRECTOR OF CLINICAL INNOVATION, CAREQUEST
AND FOUNDER, DR. KEEPER'S DENTAL WELLNESS

"What the World Needs Right Now"

"What the world needs right now is a one stop, self-care guide that everyone can understand. As a dental health educator and practitioner, I thank God for Dr. Phillips and her simple and effective mouth care system. Ellie Phillips has devoted herself to helping our missionary team modify her system—and explore how we could adapt it to be useful in impoverished areas of the world, where dental care is neither available or affordable. What an inspiration she is to our team!"

GERRY BEAUCHEMIN, LICENSED DENTAL THERAPIST,
DIRECTOR, DENTAL CARE FOR ALL INTERNATIONAL,
AND INVENTOR OF "GENTLE HAND-BURS"

To Walter Cooper, PhD,
for caring to ask, listen,
and encourage.

Contents

Acknowledgments

I am so honored to have Dr. Corky Willhite write the *Foreword* for this book. Dr. Willhite is the Clinical Assistant Professor, Department of Prosthodontics, LSU School of Dentistry and Faculty at the Center for Esthetic Excellence in Chicago. He is also the owner of a private practice that has been limited to cosmetic dentistry for over 30 years, during which time he has built a reputation providing the highest-quality treatments and creating wonderful smiles, while specifically striving to have these restorations last as long as possible.

During the 1990s, I attended several of Dr. Willhite's lectures at the University of Rochester, New York, and after the seminars he was always gracious and found time to discuss the overlooked impact of mouth acidity and preventive strategies. Few dentists would have been prepared to consider and listen, but this was how our professional friendship began. For his courteous and always open-minded support, I remain deeply grateful.

It took twelve years from the day an idea entered my mind to the completion of the first edition of *Kiss Your Dentist Goodbye*, which landed in bookstores in 2008. This second edition has taken less time to prepare but it has posed entirely new challenges in terms of overall flow and presentation. The result of these efforts is the book you now have in your hand, and there are many wonderful people I wish to thank for helping me reach this goal.

There is personal coach Judy-Lee Chen Sang of Landmark Worldwide for her wisdom and understanding even as this journey began, together with the consistent guidance and encouragement that has been so kindly provided by Square One Publishers' experienced editor Anthony Pomes and respected publisher Rudy Shur. They recognized the potential for a concise yet more expansive, and simplified yet more descriptive second edition. I remain grateful for their repeated aid and stewardship in helping me to reach this exciting moment.

I also wish to thank my daughters Chrissie and Lauren, who have remained inspirational coaches along the way. At other times, my son John-Paul ("JP") and daughter Holly helpfully answered those "phone a friend" calls—and my oldest daughter Suzi, who is always a voice of caring and calm, provided delicious soup and warm hugs as well.

Thanks also to hundreds of my patients, extended family members, employees, dental and non-dental friends, and followers who have also been ready to believe and support me over the years. Thanks to my social media team—Katey, Denise, Logan, Casey, Winston, Charlie, and Christopher—for your continued good humor and help every step of the way. I must *also* thank a special group, whose support and encouragement to complete this mission has been ongoing and remains priceless: Aurora, Christie, Megan, Valerie, and Laura (for their collective support at work, which gave me time necessary for writing); Anne and Helen (my best school friends from Great Britain); Judy and Bud, LuAnn, Steve, Tina, Vicky, and Stacy (all friends who have encouraged me but always ensured I had sufficient downtime on the porch or pickleball court).

Within dentistry, I have been blessed with a vibrant tribe of strong supporters—hygienists and dentists who are enthusiastic about a new era for dentistry—and these good people include: Elodie and Shelly (such savvy hygienists); Cyndee Johnson, who coaches those in dental offices how to raise productivity with preventive education and xylitol; Dr. Steve Edwards, an entrepreneur for the past twenty years (and counting) who is passionate about oral fitness and always adds a friendly "like" to my LinkedIn posts; Dr. Chris Kammer, who is on a similar mission to limit unnecessary treatments and educate patients about the importance of oral health; Dr. Ameet Trivedi, an outspoken dentist on social media; Donna Crawford, a health expert who supported my system of care in the nitric oxide world (when many mouthwash myths were still prevalent); Dr. Spencer Wood, a champion for new ideas and professional networking; Dr. Quinn Yost, a vibrant pediatric dentist blazing a trail in California; and also, Sarah Luetki together with Dr. Christine Hao, two dedicated professionals who operate "Sound Care" mobile units for elderly and disabled patients—and who have created a website for patients to access testimonial-driven preventive care providers.

The world of minimally invasive dentistry includes some of the finest dentists in the world, some of whom you will read about in this book, particularly in the sections that discuss xylitol or the no-drill Atraumatic Restorative Technique (ART) that is gradually being offered in more dental offices worldwide. Some of these fine professionals include dental therapist and mission caregivers Gerry Beauchemin and Jason Padvorac. Also in this group are highly respected educators, thought leaders, dentists, and doctors including: Dr. John Frachella, Dr. Jeremy Horst, Dr. Peter Milgrom, Dr. Eva Soderling, Dr. Greg Valentine, Dr. Brad Bale, and Dr. Amy Doneen. Thank you all for your professional friendship, expertise, and enthusiasm for our shared mission.

I could never have become a dentist without the scientific education offered by the prestigious Cheltenham Ladies College in England. Back in the day, I found out firsthand that women were only welcomed into the male-dominated world of medicine if they achieved the highest grades in chemistry, biology, physics, and Latin. This scientific basis inspired me to delve deeper into the biochemistry of oral health and be encouraged by other free spirits, throughout history, who dared to veer from the well-trodden pathway with new ideas about health and wellness. And so, I send my thanks to all those great minds as well. We have come a long way . . .

$\mathcal{F}$oreword

Only in the last few years have I come to appreciate the fact that I was missing an important component for ultimate patient care—the underlying balance of a patient's oral health. Whenever I can convince my patients to follow the simple steps that my trusted colleague and friend Dr. Ellie recommends, both through her patient education coaching and in the pages of this book that you are now reading, I'm confident that the dentistry in their mouths will last longer and is more likely to be a permanent solution for their lifetime.

Checking the insurance industry records of treatments performed each year continues to reveal that people of *all* ages—children, teens, young adults, middle-agers, and senior citizens alike—struggle with expensive and invasive dental problems that can affect their physical and mental health in damaging ways. This is an unacceptable outcome and anyone who cares about their oral health should be able to learn how to avoid being one more of these scary statistics—and this is why I am delighted about this fully revised second edition of Dr. Ellie's longtime bestseller. I feel certain, beyond a doubt, that this wonderfully ambitious new book will empower those in search of useful dental knowledge and relevant answers to questions about so many confusing oral care issues.

The first edition of *Kiss Your Dentist Goodbye* challenged us to stop believing that sugar was the only culprit in dental disease—and consider the idea that acidity should take more of the blame. Now, in this new second edition, Dr. Ellie weaves this knowledge together with an understanding of oral bacteria and layers it with the impact of mouth resting, xylitol, and the effect of nutrition on the microbiological ecology in our mouths. It feels to me as if this new book will move forward the understanding of experts and laypersons when it comes to maintaining healthier teeth and gums. So, here's to Dr. Ellie's ongoing and brave new work, which I believe will continue to create positive change in the world of dentists and dentistry—and, of course, in the lives of so many people worldwide.

—**Corky Willhite, DDS**
Accredited Fellow, American Academy of Cosmetic Dentistry (AACD),
Owner, the Smile Design Center, private practice limited to
cosmetic dentistry, New Orleans, LA

$\mathscr{P}$reface

The great thing in this world is not so much where we are,
but in what direction we are moving.
—OLIVER WENDELL HOLMES, SR.

I f you are concerned about tooth care, you are not alone. As a native
Brit, my dental career has unfurled between two continents—first
in Europe, and then North America. Working on both sides of the
Atlantic, I have gradually recognized a stark contrast in dental care—
with dentists and access to dental offices touted as an apparent necessity for oral health in America, whereas a reliance on natural healing,
diet, and the use of xylitol appears to deliver effective prevention
to minimize dental needs in many European countries. Dentistry in
North America has experienced amazing technological progress in
recent years. For patients to be adequately empowered to make good
decisions about their treatment needs, however, we need to recognize and unpack a large amount of mouth health knowledge that has
been ignored by professionals and misunderstood by laypersons for
over a century.

Much of my early motivation in helping people care for their
teeth came from my own family's unfortunate dental health experiences. Looking back at most formal dental school training programs
on both sides of the Atlantic shows glaring omissions within the
science of *why* people suffer tooth loss, gum disease, and cavities.
Even today in dental offices worldwide, the blame is unfairly placed

on two habits that are directly under a patient's individual control—either too much candy, or poor tooth brushing and flossing habits. In my family, however, I knew that my own parents rarely ate sweets and were meticulous about oral hygiene—and yet they both suffered severe cavities and gum disease.

My father had all his teeth extracted and replaced with dentures at the age of 35, a military strategy that assured soldiers would avoid dental problems on the battlefield. Likewise, my mother was told when she was 45 years old that she would need to have the same procedure that my father had undergone. Her diagnosis came at a time when I was studying at Guy's Hospital Dental School in London, in the Preventive Dentistry department. Back then, there were no dentists specializing in gum or periodontal disease in the UK and very few hygienists, so it was the *general* dentists who were instead trained to clean patients' teeth and perform the gum surgery known as a *gingivectomy*.

This surgery involved cutting and stitching a patient's gums, so as to try and tighten them in an often-futile attempt to prevent the tooth—or teeth—from falling out. It seemed obvious to any observant student that these efforts only led to pain, disfigurement—and to a somewhat delayed but *eventual* tooth loss. This was not the treatment I recommended to my mother, but there were more reasons why I wanted to help my mother find a different—and *better*—option to overcome gum disease and keep her natural teeth intact for life.

In the 1960s, an initial study had been published about the oral, general, and mental health of nuns living in a convent. The final study that followed spanned several decades and confirmed a concerning correlation between early full-mouth tooth extraction in these women with an increased risk of dementia. Given my own family's experiences with early-onset dementia, I implored my mother to avoid full-mouth extractions, to refuse a gingivectomy, and to instead let me find the best way for her to care for her teeth at home. This was how I came to create and develop a basic system of over-the-counter mouth rinses that she could use—and the results were nothing short of remarkable. Not only did she evade early-onset dementia, but she also maintained healthy, disease-free teeth for the next fifty years until her passing at age 95. Being able to help my mother as I had not only expanded my practical knowledge about the value of *home* daily dental care for effective disease prevention, but also instilled in me a confidence in the belief that every individual has the power to stop, prevent, and even reverse dental problems by *themselves.*

When it comes to doing things a little differently in the world of dentistry, I have noticed that being open to new ideas often depends on having a history of diverse clinical *experiences*—perhaps even more than from a prolonged academic education or beliefs derived from so-called *scientific* study results. Most of us have watched as scientific studies are overturned by new information and understanding. Personally, I was blessed with the benefit of working in three different countries—and learning important lessons in each place.

Soon after I graduated from Guy's Hospital Medical School, I began work as a dentist in Lausanne, Switzerland. It was there where I noticed that the majority of the patients that I saw enjoyed consistent oral health without the need to have repeated fluoride treatments, to drink fluoridated water, or to floss. I came to understand that the fine quality of their teeth had *everything* to do with nutrition and eating patterns, ending every meal with some kind of tooth-protective food. Additionally, it was under the guidance of my Swiss counterpart that I learned how gum massage could restore gum health. Armed with these formative experiences, I returned to England and opened my own preventive dental office in the resort town of Eastbourne. It was there that I built my practice—teaching patients everything I knew about the science of oral care.

By the end of 1980 I had a large and loyal following of patients in the UK, nearly all of whom had achieved sustainable oral health without the need for ongoing dental treatments—and many finding that even periodic cleanings became less necessary. Family responsibilities led me to leave my practice in Eastbourne, though, and relocate to Rochester, New York. Now that I was working in the US, I specialized in pediatric dentistry and became the outpatient clinic director at the Eastman Institute for Oral Health. In this capacity, I was fortunate to work alongside a professor whose career had been steeped in the research of *xylitol*. A unique and delicious sugar derived from plant sources, xylitol has been used for decades in Switzerland, Finland, and *elsewhere* throughout Europe to support general and oral health. Xylitol—when used frequently and *appropriately*—can actively help to prevent cavities and improve overall gum and tooth health.

Something to Think About

Please understand that this book is *not* meant to criticize or wantonly demonize the dental profession, or the professionals who care for you during dental visits. Its purpose instead is to share the latest scientific knowledge and equip you with strategies that allow you to take control of your oral health and defend your teeth from damage and disease—and to do so every day of your life. Understanding the new and ever-growing science surrounding mouth bacteria will revolutionize your view of what it means to have clean teeth, and your approach to traditional treatments and routine dentistry. However, it *all* begins with valuing your mouth health and embracing the *natural* healing capabilities of your mouth. By adopting these principles and utilizing the information in this book, you will discover effective and empowering ways to improve the condition of your teeth and gums.

Armed with a fuller understanding of xylitol and my experiences in prevention prior to my arrival in America, I was eager to share this knowledge with fellow dentists and patients alike. The science of preventing and reversing tooth decay was just becoming recognized in the US and was taught as a system called: Caries Management by Risk Assessment (CAMBRA). Spearheaded by Dr. John Featherstone, the Dean of the University of San Francisco, the CAMBRA movement resonated with me deeply. Dr. Featherstone—along with the US Surgeon General at the time, Dr. Richard Carmona—recognized the importance of disseminating this kind of preventive scientific knowledge to the public, and this has always been my passion. The encouragement and inspiration from these two professionals, with support and interest from many other dental and medical practitioners, led me to pen and then publish the first edition of this book.

For decades, I have been amazed by the remarkable capabilities of my at-home system to sustain oral health, remineralize teeth, and help to reverse and heal cavities and gum disease. The universality of this system's ability to address gum disease and cavities has always interested and excited me. Also, it works for all ages, for men and women, for anyone young or old with adult teeth who is able and willing to use a specific sequence of mouth rinses and toothpaste in the method I recommend. Talking with my patients showed me what many studies had begun to illustrate—a connection between oral, digestive and systemic, whole-body health. Patients using my system had noticed on tests that their body inflammation was improving, *without medication*. This is why I helped to create the American Academy for Oral Systemic Health (AAOSH), a not-for-profit organization dedicated to sharing science and information linking systemic with oral health.

I have watched with joy as the oral care system that I developed—and which you will learn about in greater depth throughout this book—became a staple for my family, friends, and countless patients over the years. Incredible numbers of people have followed this system faithfully for decades and have marveled at the results, as their oral health improved, and they witnessed cavities and gum disease heal and often completely reverse. These fortunate individuals have experienced years of sustainable oral health—and still today maintain a cavity-free mouth and healthy gums.

The excitement surrounding this system remains palpable since the release of my first edition of *Kiss Your Dentist Goodbye*. Yet, since the book's publication, the awful statistics of cavities that occur in young children and adolescent teeth—along with overall costs for office cleanings, X-rays, fillings, implants, surgeries, and gum treatments for young and old alike—continue to escalate. Drawing from the information in this newly revised and fully updated Second Edition, readers across the globe—and parents in *particular*—will now be able to take charge of their family's oral health and offer children the oral health protection that can give them a future with fewer dental problems or need for interventions. This book explains the easy strategies that will *bring* this rapid improvement in oral health, and will empower you to ultimately limit all unnecessary dental treatments and expenses—for *life*.

$\mathcal{I}$ntroduction

Natural forces within us are the true healers of disease.

—HIPPOCRATES

For most of us, the process is the same. You do your best each day to take care of your teeth and gums—only to learn at your next dental visit that you once again have new cavities, that your gums are bleeding, or (worse yet) have become infected. Meanwhile, there are also people you know who seem to *never* have a problem with their teeth. If you happen to ask them for the secret to their success, chances are that they don't give their teeth much thought and cannot even tell you about specific things they have done. Frustrating? *Certainly.*

When it comes to overall success with dental care, there seems to be little fairness in the equation. Why does it cost you an arm and a leg each time you or your kids go to a dentist, while these other lucky people simply have check-ups and are done? Is it their good genes? Is it because of the water they drink? Or is it perhaps just a case of good—or bad—karma?

For years, we have been told to take care of our teeth by brushing and flossing. And yet, the majority of American adults by age sixty-five find themselves in constant need of fillings, dental repairs, crowns, and cleanings that seem to get progressively more expensive and complicated no matter how often they visit a dentist. What is it that these other folks are doing right, and that the rest of us seem to be doing *wrong*? These are important questions, and they just illustrate

1

how complex tooth care can be for most people. This book has been designed to make oral care easily understandable and explain how to take control of your mouth health and feel more empowered so that you can avoid unnecessary dental treatments, cavities, and the dangers of gum disease.

As a longtime dental professional and author of this book, my role is twofold. I am here to open your eyes to the most effective oral health strategies and information available, gleaned from decades of research data and combined with years of experience observing patients in a plethora of clinical settings. Perhaps the most important help I can offer has to do with home care remedies and professional treatments that I believe you should *avoid*. At the same time, I recognize the fact that many of you who have picked up this book are *not* dental experts—and are, therefore, in need of guidance explained in a way that is easy to understand and from which one can benefit sooner rather than later. That is why we will begin with the ABCs of oral health, after which I will then break down and describe in detail the amazing, long-time oral care system that I recommend.

The first part of this book, as mentioned above, will be a primer on the basics of how teeth become damaged and how the mouth, gums, and teeth can heal. We begin with a short history of how dentistry has evolved over the ages, since the first recorded dental treatment in Egypt at the time of the Pharaohs and how things have progressed to the present day. Next, we will explore key mouth troubles that people experience—from plaque buildup, tooth wear, cavities, gum recession, swelling, yellowing teeth, and mouth sensitivity—presented alongside a simple discussion of how to keep your mouth in a state of consistent balance and health. Special attention will also be given to the incredible value of the mouth's saliva, and how it serves as a crucial determinant of mouth health. I will introduce and clarify the various things that can go wrong with teeth at any given point in life, and how poor mouth health can drastically impact the overall health and lives of adults and children alike.

After this overview of these common problems and "tooth topics," I will share the strategies that have helped many thousands of patients, friends, family, and followers around the world to become empowered when it comes to their dental health. How great it is that the usual "process" has shifted, so that people can now sit down in the dentist's chair with confidence and say "Ah"—just as their dental professionals puzzle over how dramatically their patients' oral health improved, and why they no longer need ongoing treatments or dental cleanings.

Part Two of this book will be focused tightly on my "Do-It-Yourself" system of oral care for your teeth and gums. Each element of this method can help you achieve a healthier mouth, and the way this happens will be defined and *explained* in a deliberate "step by step" fashion. My system is tailormade for both adults and children with adult teeth, and I emphasize—through both analysis and anecdote—how important it is to start this strategy as early in life as possible. Next follows an in-depth exploration of the naturally occurring health sugar known as xylitol, a product that is a cornerstone of this strategy for effective preventive care.

Also sprinkled throughout the book are a handful of informative insets that touch on various topics, including:

- Why some toothbrushes help more than others

- The all-too-real fear many of us have when going to the dentist

- The difference between treating a cavity and having your teeth cleaned at the dentist, compared with an effective home care strategy that can help you to avoid cavities and prevent gum disease

Many people are aware that lifestyle changes can improve general health, but few have considered that there are similar habits and ideas that can boost your mouth health. I recommend a few lifestyle modifications that can be used in tandem with my Complete Mouth Care System™. This can be found in a section dedicated to what I call the "Four Keys of Health" for optimal mouth care, which includes:

1. The establishment of a consistent, practical, and effective Oral Care Routine;

2. The importance of Your Mouth's Own Saliva in maintaining healthier teeth and gums;

3. The pivotal importance for you and your family to adopt healthy habits and to make educated Lifestyle Choices and Daily Habits;

   and

4. The self-regard and protective treatment of your own body's immune system as A Healing Machine, with a focus on the need for probiotics, prebiotics, and overall dietary supplementation wherein your body's own continual repair leads to a stronger and more consistent prevention of mouth disease.

After the book's *Conclusion*, readers can also consult a *Glossary* of specialized terms that you may have heard being used at a dental office during examination and/or treatment.

As you witness the impact you can have on your oral health, your relationship with your dentist will most likely evolve. Dentists excel at identifying visible signs of the invisible bacterial imbalance in our mouths, such as cavities and gum damage. Your new objective will be to use dental visits to help you to periodically evaluate your oral health, and that of your family. You may consider selecting a dentist who offers advanced diagnostic tools, comprehensive bacterial testing, and personalized protocols beyond the standard "cleaning, X-rays, and probing" approach. Armed with the knowledge provided in this book, you will be able to weigh for yourself the consequences of dental treatments and to make more informed decisions about fillings, sealants, fluoride treatments, and cleanings than ever before. Keeping a record of your progress over time can only *enhance* your understanding of the remarkable home care strategies that I will teach you about in the pages to come.

So, let this journey into a new world of oral health help make your future dental visits more intriguing, helpful, and rewarding. You have nothing to lose by taking this first step—except, of course, a lot of unnecessary treatments, expense, inconvenience, and time in the dental chair.

———

PART ONE

The Building Blocks of Better Mouth Care

1

The Dentistry Dilemma— One Step Forward, Three Steps Back?

Time is relative; its only worth depends upon what we do as it is passing.

—ALBERT EINSTEIN

While it is true that dentists excel at addressing cavities and gum disease, it is also the case that most do not know any ways to halt these ongoing dental issues or to confidently prevent or reverse these common dental problems for their patients. The current approach from dentistry can be frustratingly one-dimensional and short-sighted, as they keep focused largely on continual and periodic repair of existing problems and fixing acute damage as presented to them on each visit. Many laypersons believe—*mistakenly*—that once a cavity is fixed, the decay problem has been solved. Similarly, dental cleanings are often wrongly viewed as the best way to fight cavities. Both assumptions can lead those searching for better oral health far astray of their goal.

My experience over the years has proved to me that a good number of oral health practitioners rely on well-marketed and seemingly plausible explanations to justify ongoing dental problems to their concerned patients. I consider these so-called "explanations" as something else—I see them as convenient *excuses*. These excuses lack scientific evidence and can be harmful because they divert attention away from the actual and underlying causes of dental disease. False narratives have pervaded dentistry for decades, and many dentists seem to still believe them. Only by having the confidence to reject wrong ideas—for example, the erroneous concept that your toothbrushing is causing gum or enamel damage—will a deeper investigation then reveal that an acidic mouth, a reduced flow of saliva, or some kind of breathing obstruction may be far more likely the *real* reasons behind such maladies as tooth erosion, gum diseases and recession, plaque, cavities, or the need for repeated fillings and treatments, tooth sensitivity, and discoloration. Without defining the factors that really underlie these dental problems, the longer they will remain unaddressed, and the less chance you have of determining a remedy that will be able to control, prevent, or reverse them.

When you ask your dentist why you have cavities, enamel wear, sensitivity, or gum disease, a good percentage of patients will likely be told that *they* are to blame for their problems. Common allegations include: incorrect or insufficient flossing; aggressive brushing or not using an electric toothbrush; and tooth clenching or grinding. There is a condition called *bruxism*, which is why an accurate diagnosis is important, because this more serious kind of tooth clenching can be associated with a breathing or airway blockage, and in this case, you should be working with an airway specialist.

Catch-all explanations are *fundamentally* directed at the wrong target—at the symptom and not the *cause*. This is why so many dentists are bewildered by how to prevent or stop dental disease and damage, and why their only remedy is to treat the symptom. But your hope lies in something that you can do for yourself: take the time to try and figure out the underlying conditions of *mouth acidity* or *dryness*—the real causes of most dental problems and the primary reason why your mouth bacteria or chemistry is out of balance, creating the conditions for plaque to form, enamel to erode, or gum disease to occur. There is, without doubt, an unfortunate consequence of missing the diagnostic target, as patients need to return over and over for ongoing office therapies. But if you address the actual cause of these problems, they normally resolve in a shockingly rapid fashion, and this will put an end to those progressive, often never-ending dental treatments.

This shift in thinking appears to be the fatal flaw at the heart of modern dental practice—and as we step forward with new dental treatment modalities, we are at risk for taking the proverbial "three steps back" and missing the very thing that helps patients achieve what she or he truly wants—less treatment and a simple way to enjoy healthy teeth and gums.

Only through a blended approach—mixing equal parts of scientific knowledge, clinical observation, and some kind of a standardized method of *oral health assessment*—will we uncover the best ways to prevent dental problems and limit unnecessary dental treatments. Until this occurs, it is only with an accurate diagnosis (or discovering the real *reason* for dental problems), that patients will be able to select the correct strategies tailored to prevent, improve, and even reverse those specific problems. To understand why this is not how mainstream dentistry operates today, it may be helpful to look at how dentistry evolved over its one-hundred-year history—and examine how, and *why*, ideas from the past continue to cause confusion and antagonism within the profession to the present day.

Examples of this include the supporters and dissenters on topics such as the impact of a dead tooth on general health, the risks and benefits of fluoride, those who believe silver fillings and root canals are toxic, and others who decry implants or warn of harm from home-care toothpaste and mouth rinsing. Some of these subjects cause friendly animosity, but others have caused division and hostility within dentistry and a split in the profession. The result is that patients can feel confused and lack trust, often stirred by mischievous marketing, financial interests, and chatter on social media. On these controversial topics, I find myself on challenging but interesting "middle ground," which may be the result of my long and diverse clinical experiences, my opportunities to learn about decay prevention and gum disease from world-renown researchers, from treating patients in high-risk communities, or by being exposed to the recent and evolving science of the oral microbiome. So, let's look back at the history of dentistry to understand how this colorful palette of dental ideas originated and developed over time.

DENTISTRY OF *YESTERDAY*

As far back as recorded time reveals, oral health care has stood as a basic and consistent part of the human story. Before the modern-day advent of commercially sold toothbrushes and toothpastes, many cultures across the globe have made successful use of various natural sticks and powders to help keep their teeth and gums clean. Indeed, the origins of dentistry can be *first* traced back thousands of years to the time of the Third Dynasty of Egypt circa 2686–2613 BCE (Before Common Era). This was the period when an early physician known as Hesy-Ra was recorded as treating Egyptian citizens for problems with their teeth.

Just as important as the first evidence of dental care are the tools that have been used to keep teeth strong and healthy. Take, for example, the Miswak stick. This twig (or root cutting) is trimmed from what is known as the "toothbrush tree" (*Salvadora persica*), and the Miswak stick has been (and is *still*) used as a natural mouth care tool to clean the teeth and massage the gums in many countries around the world—particularly the Middle East regions and across the continent of Africa.

The ends of these wooden *sticks* are purposely shredded and frayed to create a small brush that is used to massage the gums. To avoid transmitting infection, this brush is maintained regularly by clipping the end, to remove any worn or infected bristles. The Miswak stick contains compounds that stimulate saliva flow and provide essentials oils, minerals, silica (a common mineral in the earth's crust), and even *fluoride*. The Mizwak stick has thousands of years of history and studies to illustrate its positive benefits. Today, the Mizwak is readily available online and its use may be of interest to some patients and dentists as an effective strategy for travel and in other specific situations.

Similar tools for dental care were known to the indigenous people of North America to be cut from birch trees. Many simple but effective remedies have emerged throughout history and a natural approach to oral well-being is appealing. This stands in contrast to a treatment-centered dental approach that appears to have its origins in the early 1300s. At this time, people in the Western world generally showed little interest in the personal care of their teeth. They usually relied on others to deal with any dental problems that arose. Without daily care, many people suffered from dental decay and the consequences of rotten teeth.

Dentistry's solution was treatment that mainly involved tooth extraction. This kind of dentistry was performed by the medieval "barber surgeons" who used crude forcep-like instruments to do the job. In the 1700s, a particularly aggressive "door key" tool became popular, used to loosen and extract diseased and damaged teeth from patients' mouths. Since dental anesthetics like lidocaine and procaine were not used in dentistry until the early 1900s, dental treatment of this era must have been extremely traumatic and unpleasant.

As mentioned, there has been a long history of oral care, long before the invention of the toothbrush, forceps, or tooth keys. The indigenous people of North America used a form of "chew stick" fashioned from a white-barked birch tree that grows in many colder climates, especially in North America, Scandinavia, and in northern parts of Turkey, Russia, and China. Birch-derived sticks were used to clean teeth and found to naturally promote and maintain oral health. Within the fibers of this wood is a sugar called *xylitol*. (We will discuss *xylitol* in greater detail in Part Two of this book.) With the help of these sticks, users were able to stimulate saliva and prevent plaque buildup in the mouth. Even today, children in parts of Russia and Scandinavia are trained to rinse their teeth with the sap from birch trees, and in Finland, there are public health programs to supply daily xylitol in chewing gum to preschool children across the country. In Turkey and China, it is common to chew xylitol gum and

Getting a Handle on the Toothbrush

Though there exist similarly structured antecedents dating back to 3500 BCE in Egypt, the earliest invention of the tool that today we recognize as the *toothbrush* dates to early seventh-century China during the Tang Dynasty. Its initial design stemmed from a small bunch of hog hair bristles attached to a sturdy handle made from wood or bone. These preliminary brushes were further refined in design when they were first introduced to Europe during the seventeenth century. Manufactured brushes began to be produced in the 1780s, and although this may seem like progress for dentistry, it was perhaps the tool responsible for leading us into a dental backslide. These new brushes were merely wooden sticks with coarse pig hair or beaver bristles attached at the head—and, as it turned out, they easily picked up bacteria.

Many people shared the same toothbrush, which would have caused a spreading of the bacterial infection that grows plaque and causes dental disease. Perhaps the invention of the toothbrush has caused *more* dental disease than it has solved. Of course, at this same time in the Western world, communities began to have easier access to less expensive and more refined grains and sugars, which likely exacerbated the rampant problems of dental decay and gum disease.

The toothbrush was progressively improved in design, and one with three distinct rows of brushes became popular after its introduction in 1844. By the late 1930s, rough animal-hair bristles were replaced with nylon and produced internationally by Dupont de Nemours—to create Doctor West's Miracle Toothbrush, which was introduced to the marketplace with excitement.

By the 1950s, the advent of television advertising generated surprising interest in home care products and a toothpaste called Pepsodent. Many companies experimented with ingredients and their formulations of toothpaste. By this time, there had been the discovery of the mineral fluoride in certain water supplies in areas of America and later it was found to have a relationship with lower risk for cavities. The first company to run clinical trials and prove the benefits of fluoride toothpaste was Crest. This was also the time when the world had entered the Space Age, and many new technologies were emerging, including the Squibb Corporation (who later merged in 1989 with Bristol-Myers to become one of the biggest pharmaceutical companies in the world) and who were first to introduce an electric toothbrush—known as the "Broxodent."

The 1970s was a time when sugar was believed to cause cavities and food particles were believed to cause gum disease. A toothbrush with a single row of bristles was suggested and the technique was to hold the brush below the gum line at a specific angle. This Dr. Bass brush and brushing technique is still recommended by some dentists today, but there are problems with it—particularly since the benefits of gum massage are now more commonly recognized, and a brush with *more* bristles is seen as the more effective method for this approach. For adequate tooth cleaning and massage, we need a brush with a dense bristlehead, although now the problem is that disease bacteria can multiply and become more aggressive in the low-oxygen conditions among the dense bristles. Toothbrushes require good disinfection, and it's a good idea to completely dry a toothbrush between each use to help prevent problems. In addition, it is always a helpful idea to replace a current toothbrush with an as-yet-unused one on a consistent and periodic basis. While the frequency with which you swap out the old for the new is ultimately up to you, a generally decent rule of thumb would be once a month.

By the turn of the twenty-first century, the toothbrush had evolved to the point where battery-driven oscillating brushes were marketed as the best way to keep teeth clean and gleaming white, selling the ideas with unrealistic animations of how the brush cleans your teeth. Today, there are even more ideas and designs, some using Bluetooth-compatible technology, to track daily brushing habits through a digital app owned by the manufacturing companies. Even with all these advances and technology, the incidence of gum disease is on the rise and cavities are just as problematic as they have ever been for children and adults of all ages. This explains why we need to look beyond toothbrushes and toothpaste and uncover what is the real underlying cause of dental problems. As we have begun to realize at this point across all levels of life and culture, increases in technological refinement and know-how mean next to nothing if not paired with the wisdom that comes from *knowledge.* To be best equipped to handle oral health issues, one must understand the subject at its core. Then we will be able to stop, prevent, and reverse dental disease—forever.

gain protection from plaque and decay. However, while the value of xylitol has been recognized in many parts of Europe, it has not yet been fully recognized or appreciated by the profession of dentistry in the US or across the British Isles.

There have, of course, been numerous discoveries and amazing changes that have impacted dentistry in positive ways, especially in the field of cosmetic restorations and the work that helps patients keep a nice full smile. In the mid-1800s, for instance, dentistry began to offer more comprehensive services and help people avoid the need for extractions. These services included tooth repairs, fillings and, if necessary, some kind of replacement for lost teeth. It was during this time that an English chemist named Dr. Joseph Bell introduced *amalgam*, an inorganic mercury-based material used to fill cavities in teeth.

Here again, the advancement came at a cost. At the time of its introduction, there was a loud outcry from doctors and dentists about the mercury content in this filling material. Mercury was known to have negative effects on human health, and mercury poisoning was known within the medical profession as *erethism*. The damage from mercury had already been noticed and examined among workers in the hat-making industry, where it had been found to cause lasting neurological damage. In fact, the "Mad Hatter" character from legendary English author Lewis Carroll's iconic 1865 novel *Alice's Adventures in Wonderland* was a satiric reference to the problems that had been discovered from mercury poisoning.

Despite the many concerns, enough dentists wanted to use amalgam and were excited about its affordability when compared with the only other alternative of the time—gold fillings. As dental organizations debated the use of amalgam, the American Dental Association (ADA) emerged in 1859 as a "pro-amalgam" group established in Niagara Falls, New York—and which has continued to exist, and thrive, into the present day.

As amalgam fillings were introduced and the ADA was starting to become a dental force in the US, a remarkable figure from Hungary named Dr. Ignaz Semmelweis emerged in Vienna. Dr. Semmelweis proposed a theory that would eventually impact us *all*—he believed that handwashing could reduce the spread of infection. *Childbed fever* was a deadly disease that was killing many mothers and infants during childbirth. Driven by his belief that better hand hygiene for physicians amid child deliveries could save lives, Semmelweis fought all the opposing views of the medical establishment.

Only after Semmelweis' death in 1865 did German scientist August Köhler invent the modern microscope (in 1893) and prove what Dr. Semmelweis had only been able to demonstrate through conjecture and observation. The microscope established visually that bacteria were indeed transferred to others through contact during the birthing process. Finally, scientific tools were able to show the accuracy of the clinical observations of Dr. Semmelweis, which challenged the understanding of the medical profession at the turn of the century.

Semmelweis was not the first person, though, to find a connection between microorganisms and the clinical symptoms of disease. Indeed, the notion that "invisible" germs can damage one's health can be traced back in time to the Roman scholar Marcus Varro, who lived and worked in the first century BCE. Nearly five hundred years later, at the start of the Middle Ages, this idea gained wider acceptance and a millennium later, in the sixteenth century, the basic contagion theory is found mentioned in Italian, German, and French medical textbooks. Then, by the mid-nineteenth century, renowned scientific figures like French chemist Louis Pasteur, British surgeon Joseph Lister, and German microbiologist Robert Koch brought renewed attention to the idea that microorganisms can cause disease. Today, we know that bacteria can be both good and bad—with some that are essential to promote health, while others harm us—and yet, most dental schools continue to ignore this underlying mouth biology and focus almost exclusively on treatment of the resulting symptoms.

Another crucial mouth care development to take place in the nineteenth century was first introduced by an inventive dentist named G. V. Black. Dr. Black revolutionized dental practices by inventing an electric, cord-driven foot engine to power dental drills. He went on to create and document what he perceived as the ideal method for filling teeth. He standardized the formula for mixing amalgam for these fillings, created a manual of dental terminology, introduced nitrous oxide (known also as "laughing gas") for anesthesia, and recognized the damaging effects of acidity on teeth.

During a visit in the early 1900s to the city of Colorado Springs in Colorado, he crossed paths with American dentist Dr. Frederick S. McKay, soon to be known for his own pioneering fluoride research. Surprisingly, despite his obvious love of mechanics, Dr. Black was so impressed by what he learned in Colorado Springs that it changed his vision for the future of dentistry. This was expressed during a speech in 1900, foreseeing a shift toward preventive care, saying, "The day is surely coming . . . when we will be engaged in practicing preventive, rather than reparative, dentistry."

In these modern times, Dr. Black would likely question why dental decay has remained such a prevalent issue—and why the national spending for fillings and dental repairs continues to soar, exceeding $162 billion dollars in the United States in the year 2021 alone. On the other hand, Dr. Black firmly believed in dentistry's independence from medicine, and it was at this juncture that the professions began to diverge, starting to specialize in their respective areas of the body. After all, the advent of the microscope alongside the development of pharmaceuticals to control infections marked a new era for medicine, reducing the need for many surgical interventions and the risks of disfigurement associated with amputations that had previously been used to control progressive infection.

What about dentistry, though? Going back to this same era, dentistry looked for an antibiotic or vaccine solution to control the progression of cavities but was never able to establish any kind of effective therapy. Filling teeth was the preferred option to extraction, even though many physicians raised concerns about the health consequences of filling diseased teeth and the use of mercury in silver amalgam fillings. There was also the belief that an infected tooth could become a primary source of infection elsewhere in the body. The notion that was popular in the early 1900s was that a diseased tooth could affect overall body health. This was known as the

Focus of Infection theory—and although it gained attention for a time, the idea was generally ridiculed and eventually fell from favor in the 1940s.

The rift between conventional medicine and dentistry in the Western world deepened progressively over the years and the two separate professions have focused in an almost blinkered way, viewing only the importance of their own specific areas of expertise. This professional divide resulted in a lack of communication and limited understanding of the impact that poor oral health has on a patient's overall well-being. Just as most people throughout the world know that handwashing is an accepted practice to reduce disease transmission, it was not until the twentieth century before dentists even began to adequately sterilize their instruments and use disposable syringes to decrease the risks of disease transmission to patients. Another big shift occurred in 1980, when concern about the transmission of the AIDS (Acquired Immuno-Deficiency Syndrome) virus prompted dental professionals to finally wear gloves, masks, and eye protection.

Within this atmosphere of general disregard for disease transmission, ignorance about the links between oral health and medical conditions, and despite some enduring remnants of 1940s ridicule, a small group of us created an organization in 2010 that was designed to publicize the plethora of research and information linking oral health with systemic health. This organization, called the American Academy for Oral Systemic Health (AAOSH), has grown and evolved since that time, but it still struggles to find a pathway to link the medical and dental professions.

Certainly it has been able to raise awareness about the importance and value of oral health in the treatment of chronic inflammatory and other medical conditions, but there is still much work to be done to alert OB-GYN doctors about the value of xylitol to limit preterm birth, and the impact of oral health on digestive health—and in 2022, the American Academy of Periodontology showed that in a study of patients hospitalized with COVID-19 there was a correlation between poor oral health and severe COVID-19 outcomes and death.

The COVID-19 outbreak of 2020 also drew attention to other concerns within the operation of dental offices—things that for decades have been ignored as possible sources of disease transmission. Suddenly there was new interest in aerosol splatter from dental drills and tools; air quality in the dental treatment rooms; and the contamination of dental water lines, all of which are potential sources of infection and justifiable cause for concern among dental patients.

DENTISTRY OF *TODAY*—AND *TOMORROW*?

Today, we recognize the urgent need for medical and dental professionals to collaborate and address the interconnectedness between oral and systemic health. The advent of social media and increased access to information has shed further light on this issue, prompting a push for better communication. Too often doctors forget the impact of poor oral health on physical and mental health—and dentists ignore the impact of plaque, cavities, and periodontal disease on systemic health. Many also ignore the toxicity from plastics and other dental materials used in sealants, fillings, and retainers, and the fact that these plastics used in dentistry may have a long-term impact on the general health—particularly of young or high-risk patients.

While medicine has made significant advancement in educating patients about the effects of lifestyle on disease prevention and has promoted the idea of personalized risk evaluation, dentistry has remained deeply reliant on demonizing sugar and two specific treatments: tooth fillings for cavities and battling gum disease with dental cleanings. However, the Human Microbiome Project (HBP) of 2007 provided so many new insights into the importance of our oral *microbiome.*

The oral microbiome is defined, by and large, as a specific and enormous collection of microorganisms that live in the human mouth. The HBP was a lengthy study undertaken in various countries, and it showed us the importance of nurturing a healthy bacterial population in the mouth if we want to experience oral health. This is a radically new shift in perspective from the old idea that every mouth grows plaque, and we have no control over the damage that plaque causes. This revelation offers hope for the kind of preventive era in dentistry that Dr. G. V. Black spoke of back in 1900, where patients can actively manage their oral health by nurturing a healthier oral ecosystem.

By understanding a few simple things about mouth microbes, you can become your own best advocate for this preventive approach—and furthermore, you can opt to leverage personalized bacterial testing to evaluate and monitor changes in your oral health. This empowerment can allow individuals to be more proactive and to prevent the debilitating, systemic health problems that often occur in middle-age—problems we now know have associated links with poor oral health.

For a century, dentistry has promoted itself as a highly organized but reactive professional system, offering skills to identify and treat oral disease, hunting principally for any damage that has occurred since your last dental visit. Dentists and hygienists are trained to search for cavities and gum disease using tools called dental explorers, and X-rays, to detect problems. However, all these tools are designed to look for areas of weakness, decay, bone loss, and infection, and none of these tools can offer a comprehensive assessment of improvements in mouth health over time. Given the significant impact of oral health on our well-being, it's crucial we incorporate more relevant oral and general health measurements and evaluations into the routine of dental office visits.

The intricate connection between teeth and the rest of our body is far too often overlooked. Every tooth is connected to a network of blood vessels and lymphatic drainage system that extends throughout the entire body. Some of the cells inside teeth have arm-like extensions that extend into the harder section of the tooth, and these are immersed in lymphatic liquids and communicate directly with nerves that travel to the brain. It is wrong to consider teeth as indestructible objects that can be artificially whitened and bleached, drilled, and filled, sealed with plastics, and covered with metal, without causing some kind of consequence. We cannot ignore the effects of chemicals and acidity levels on our mouth's microbiome, and how vulnerable teeth and gums can be to acidity, yet healthy enamel has a strength that is harder than steel. This is why careless daily habits can impact the normal process of natural healing and lead to poor oral health and potential damage to overall body health.

Understanding the intricate relationship between oral and systemic health appears to be a vital part of the equation for those wanting to maintain a healthy lifespan. Picture your teeth not as hard inanimate structures, but rather as a sturdy coral reef, covered with delicate and easily damaged crystals. Teeth rely on the surrounding "ocean" of saliva to maintain and repair them daily. This is why saliva can both nurture or damage teeth as it interacts with them constantly—and goes on to influence their surface hardness.

Saliva quality and flow vary with a daily rhythm known as a *Circadian rhythm*, and this rhythm is affected by many things, including our eating and drinking habits. Some foods and beverages can make saliva highly acidic, eroding minerals from teeth and weakening them. Healthy saliva has the opposite effect and can quickly replenish minerals to compensate for any loss, provided that the assaults on teeth are not too frequent and occur at a time when saliva flows freely afterward. At night, when we lie down to sleep, salivary flow decreases and may stop, and this is a time when saliva usually becomes acidic, making late-night snacking or drinking particularly dangerous for dental health. This explains why the optimal time for oral care, using products that support tooth health, is right before sleeping at night, ensuring a clean and protected oral environment overnight.

As a dental student, I learned along with my colleagues that a gleaming smile and pearly white teeth were a universal symbol of overall good health and habits. But times have changed, and white teeth may no longer guarantee a healthy person is behind that smile. Often those deceivingly bright smiles are artificially whitened, masking a world of plaque and a mouth teeming with the harmful, transmissible bacteria of chronic *periodontal* gum disease. Crafty marketing campaigns have convinced almost all of us, including dentists, that tooth whitening is a safe and effective solution to improve the color of your teeth. The many negative consequences of artificial tooth whitening are dismissed, disregarded, or ignored, and in many dental offices the service is offered with great enthusiasm and gusto.

The fact is that all artificial whitening products weaken the structure of teeth, damage the tooth's outer enamel, and disrupt the tooth's outer protein protection to some degree. In addition, they can harm the mouth's healthy bacterial population, and potentially cause irreparable DNA damage to the valuable stem cells that live inside the central pulp area of adult and children's teeth. Dentists, once staunchly against whitening, have succumbed to public pressure, as everyone clamors for more brilliant, whiter teeth—with choices today that merge into the color spectrum blue, a shade that intensified the color white. Sadly, the long-term consequences of these treatments, especially if they are frequent or in younger teeth, can be very destructive, and weakened enamel can become sensitive, gums may recede, and teeth can even die or fracture.

Here's the consideration: Artificial tooth-whitening products make teeth porous, which makes enamel stain more easily and thus creates a greater risk for wear, fracture, sensitivity, and changes that loosen fillings. *Peroxide,* an active chemical ingredient in whitening products, is capable of irritating tooth nerves, particularly if you have an untreated cavity that provides an opening for the peroxide to seep deeper inside the tooth. The peroxide and acidity of these products combine to quickly strip the protective protein layer from the outside surfaces of teeth, leaving them defenseless against invasion by cavity bacteria, and at risk for enamel fracture and loss from tooth brushing or from clenching your teeth.

So, you may ask, what about those dazzling celebrity smiles that look so great? The shocking truth is that most of those perfect smiles, possibly including the smile of your own dentist, are illusions, created by veneers, cosmetic crowns, implants, and even dentures anchored to the jaw by screws and press studs. The truth behind most glamorous grins is a far cry from the beauty of a healthy and *natural* smile.

There are dentists who refuse to offer tooth whitening, and many dentists with whom I have discussed this topic share a sense of despair, being concerned that too often patient demands so frequently dictate offerings in dental offices, sometimes with complete disregard for long-term oral health. The line blurs between what constitutes inappropriately straightened teeth—all championed by the marketing machinery of the American dental industry. The corporate giants peddle not only whitening products but dental equipment, filling materials, retainers and implants, and lasers, while a parallel universe of marketing gurus and business coaches frequently guide dentists on how best to maximize their income, maneuver the insurance systems, and form lucrative alliances within the political hallways of Washington, DC. (In Part Two, we will describe the strategies that strengthen and concurrently whiten teeth *naturally*, while safeguarding our precious oral health.)

The good news is that dentists in the United States still command great respect from the public, and many patients feeling genuine affection for their dentist. The crux of the issue is not practitioners or their treatments, but rather the widespread misconceptions about the dentist's role in helping individuals achieve ultimate oral health. Today we grasp the profound impact of oral health on overall health, reaching far beyond the desire to avoid pain, preserve teeth, or remove an infected tooth. The desire is to know how to best enjoy sustainable mouth health that is known to be a necessary goal for longevity, and a way to preserve our health in our senior years. Oral health is a vital asset, capable of reducing our risk for heart attack, stroke, diabetes, arthritis, pre-term birth, digestive disorders, cognitive decline, Alzheimer's, and early-onset dementia.

The most important challenge is to create a true definition or description of what constitutes a healthy mouth. This is a formidable challenge with the rise of computer-generated crowns and veneers that have blurred the line between genuine and artificial smiles, making it difficult to discern the authenticity of a beautiful smile. How can we gauge the health of our own mouths? Straight teeth, a lack of bleeding, no cavities, or even a dentist's assurance that your mouth is healthy does not provide a definitive indication.

A healthy mouth transcends these superficial outcomes and operates in an active way, where the biology and chemistry of the mouth is balanced and ready to protect our teeth and gums by immediately repairing and healing any damage that occurs. This delicate balance empowers us to halt and prevent cavities, reduce sensitivity, heal gum problems, and safeguard any mineral loss that can lead to erosion, abrasion, or enamel weakness. When our mouths possess this capacity to swiftly reverse damage, it allows us to preserve our teeth and gums year after year for life.

If followed, this new and vibrant approach to mouth care should improve both the present and future state of dentistry—and relegate the notions of inherited dental problems, or the idea that we cannot control cavities, into the ashbin of the past . . . where they clearly belong.

2

$\mathcal{W}$atch Your Mouth— What's Visible, and Invisible, Within Our Mouths

I would not put a thief in my mouth to steal my brains.

—WILLIAM SHAKESPEARE,
THE TRAGEDY OF OTHELLO

In this chapter, my goal is to look at the human mouth—and explain the various hidden influences, and health links, that exist between the mouth and other areas of the head and neck. I will also provide an overview of the fascinating connections between the chemistry and the microorganisms that reside within our mouth, and in many adjacent and interconnected anatomical areas.

This "invisible" anatomy of the mouth is finally being better understood and appreciated. The more that we can fathom about this world of liquids and particles (which are all too small for the naked eye to see), the more we realize the crucial role they play in supporting our mouths' regenerative capabilities. Unfortunately, many individuals unknowingly damage their mouth health through their own harmful daily habits and improper oral care routines. The mouth's ability to keep itself safe has long been ignored because, in a healthy mouth, these interacting elements work harmoniously to shield our teeth and gums from any potential damage.

The problems of cavities and progressive gum disease occur when these hidden assets are absent, impaired, or have been rendered dysfunctional by our own damaging daily lifestyle choices. The connection between our mouth and the anatomy surrounding it also needs to be considered by anyone who has unsuccessfully tried to control the spread of cavities, bad breath (often called *halitosis*—please see the *Glossary* at the end of this book for a fuller definition of this term, along with many others that you will read about as we move forward), or interrelated gum and periodontal disease. The adjacent areas of the head and neck do, in fact, have great potential to support or adversely affect our oral health. So, perhaps we should begin to view the condition of our teeth and gums in a more expansive way—as being all in our heads, *literally*.

MOUTH 101—EAR, NOSE, SINUS, AND THROAT

The anatomy of the human mouth can be divided into two categories—that which is *visible* (teeth, gums, tongue, and the inner skin of the mouth) and that which I would describe, by way of comparison, as *invisible*. When it comes to our mouth, the seldom-appreciated links can be found in the connection of the mouth to the throat; and how the throat leads to the breathing tubes that travel into the lungs and also the esophagus, which then leads into the digestive tract.

There is also a less recognized, but no less direct, connection at the throat-mouth junction. This is where a part of our head's anatomy—the *Eustachian tubes*—enters into our middle ear at the back of the throat, positioned close to the entry points for the back of the nose that leads out from the sinuses and nasal passages. The sinus areas of the face and forehead regions are spaces of relative emptiness within the bones of our face—and they stretch and wind their way behind our nose and cheeks, and even into the center of our head. Ultimately, all these passageways are connected in one or more ways to the throat and therefore indirectly to the environment within our mouth.

Understanding that our mouth is connected to all these separate areas can help us look at oral health in a more expansive way. The health of one area of the head and neck can influence an adjacent area, either positively or negatively. Anyone of any age who experiences chronic cavities or gum disease should always consider their nasal and sinus health, as well as their gastric and lung health. After all, it is knowing about the linkage of these pathways—and balancing the health of so many interconnecting yet apparently different areas of the body—that can impact your personal journey toward improved and sustainable oral health.

Blood Flow to the Face and Mouth

The surprising number of blood vessels that connect our face and mouth is yet another anatomical wonder. Blood from the face, mouth, nasal passages, and sinuses circulates and eventually returns to the heart and lungs through what are called *venous* (related to the body's veins) blood vessels and—in particular—the *brachiocephalic vein*, which extends directly from the body's *thorax* (the area of the human body that rests between the neck and the abdomen—see *Glossary*) and then travels further downward to the upper right portion of the chest. In the lungs, blood is continually oxygenated and then pumped back to the face, nose, and mouth area. The venous blood vessel system from the face and mouth is especially complex, with many intercommunicating and large caliber veins that lead to small valve-less veins located on each side of our jaws. This area is called the *pterygoid plexus*. Researchers do not yet know the functions of this particular spot in the mouth, but it appears the veins are massaged by muscle movements whenever we smile, eat, or talk.

As it turns out, masses of what we call *stem cells* (a specific type of cell in the human body that can change its form to develop into any kind of new bone, skin, or gum cell—in essence, whatever the body needs to repair itself) are found on the inside walls of veins. Stem cells anywhere in the body can be stimulated by certain signals, including massage in a nearby area, to travel outside the vein walls. Once this takes place, they can flatten and curl up to create a form of *new* blood vessels, which then will carry blood for healing to an area where skin, bone, or gum tissue has been damaged. This process is called *angiogenesis*, and it is the initial step in the natural process of repair that the body puts into motion every time we cut ourselves— or when we need to grow new skin on our face or on the inside of our mouth.

The presence of so many stem cells in the blood vessels of the aforementioned *pterygoid plexus* has not yet been fully evaluated. It is interesting, however, to consider the utility of this complex blood supply to the mouth and face. Clinical experience indicates that massaging the gums with a suitable toothbrush—by brushing above and *around* the gum supporting a tooth—is precisely the type of stimulation that can help to regrow the lost gum tissue. This process likely begins with the encouragement of stem cells to form new *capillaries* (very small blood vessels), which would then carry blood for the transportation of all the necessary nutrients and materials required for gum healing.

For decades, dentists have protested that our gums cannot regrow. I suggest, however, that the stimulation of surrounding stem cells *can* in fact encourage restorative growth in this area of the mouth—through the simple process of gum massage. To achieve this outcome, patients need to use a sufficiently dense and resilient toothbrush in tandem with a good brushing technique. I have witnessed decades of clinical success stories—but in every case, the patient had to first stop damaging their gums.

This worrisome situation can unfold for a number of reasons. It can be the result of improper tooth movements during orthodontic treatments, either after teeth are straightened with braces or from the ongoing use of a preformed series of retainers that remain in common use today (known generally as *Invisalign*). The trouble can also start as a result of what are known as *night guards*. These products are plastic plates made by a dentist to protect teeth from the continual grinding that may occur while we sleep. Plastic retainers, used to prevent teeth from moving out of line, may also be the culprit. Surprisingly enough, it may even happen as a side effect of ineffective or insufficient brushing; aggressive cleaning between teeth with small cone-shaped or graded tools or brushes; or even from the harsh and excessive use of dental floss. The instructions for gum massage techniques—along with my Complete Mouth Care System™—will be described more fully in Part Two of this book.

Dental Fears

Are people naturally afraid of dentists—or is it something that is learned from the culture? For as long as the profession of dentistry has existed, there seems to have been some level of suspicion and distrust when it comes to dentistry and dental procedures. For millions of people, going to the dentist can be a major source of stress and anxiety, especially when an individual feels they have no control over their dental problems.

As with so many things, a fearfully imagined dental procedure can frequently be far from what occurs in reality. Many people develop serious dental fears early in life—often after negative experiences they may have had as young children. When I was growing up in England, it was not unusual to hear parents threaten to take a misbehaving child to the dentist as punishment. Those who have had negative dental experiences usually feel the worst anxiety. Conversely, the less treatment that you need during dental visits, the more likely those visits will be enjoyable.

This is why it is important to feel empowered, and to use effective care methods that will help you to protect your mouth, teeth, and gums from unnecessary dental treatments. Your own active participation in keeping your mouth clean and healthy will give you the best opportunity for a lifetime of happy dental visits—and sustainable oral health.

A NATURAL SYSTEM OF TOOTH REPAIR

In any discussion and exploration of the human mouth, one must never forget or overlook the crucial importance of our *teeth*—and especially the natural system of repair at play. To get a better sense of this remarkable natural process, I encourage you to consider any one of your teeth as being similar to a chicken egg—with a fiercely protective outer shell that shields the far softer parts *inside*. Maintaining the strength and integrity of this shell is paramount to preserving the health of your teeth, and this next section will provide you with a better sense of the scope and detail with which the natural elements of your mouth will help preserve those pearly whites that comprise the smile you show to the world—by fortifying the dental *strength* therein.

Welcome to the *Enamel* Kingdom

Our teeth are covered by a thin shell that we call *enamel*—this is a substance made up of crystals arranged in such a way that they provide teeth with an amazing level of protection and strength, especially considering the enamel crystals' delicate composition. Some people are surprised to learn that the outside of a tooth is so dynamic and ever-changing, but it is this specific attribute that allows enamel to maintain its enormous strength which, when healthy, protects the softer layers of *dentin* and *pulp* inside a tooth.

Dentin is a naturally occurring organic material that occupies the bulk of a tooth's mass. It is a porous layer that supports the enamel shell on the outside, while surrounding a central chamber—known in this context as the *pulp*—that is located inside every tooth. The pulp serves as the nerve center of each tooth and the home to many vital cells, nerves, and blood vessels that give life to a tooth. This area is also full of *lymph* (a clear to near-white fluid comprised of white blood cells, whose primary biologic mission is to rid the body of bacterial infection). Also within the pulp are tooth-protecting cells, with long arms that travel through the porous material of the dentin, and which also float in the lymph that fills these open spaces. These dentin cells are sensitive to any kind of tooth irritation or damage, including but not limited to: cutting with a drill; pressure from a dental tool; and they can easily initiate a pain-based reaction when they sense any pressure or temperature changes—from hot or cold air, or liquids.

For the protection of these softer and vital inner parts of a tooth, it is important for dental enamel to stay strong throughout life without any sign of aging—but this requires we care for it effectively and in a way that allows the ongoing, and *necessary*, natural repairs that cause its crystals to regenerate every day. Proper daily tooth care can assist this process and help tooth enamel to stay strong and accomplish its protective tasks throughout life.

Viewing enamel under a powerful microscope is awe-inspiring, and learning about the structure of enamel can help us better care for our teeth and perhaps see them in a new way—as a particularly exciting part of the human body. As we have already established, enamel is made up of small, hard crystals packed tightly inside the open spaces of a mesh-like scaffold that surrounds them. Small amounts of protein add resilience to enamel, supporting the delicate but hard enamel crystals that have an ability to shrink and grow, depending on the composition and acidity of the mouth liquids that surround them.

The repetitive and organized arrangement of the enamel crystals within this lattice creates the outer shell that covers and coats our teeth. The intricate but tough framework is packed with enamel crystals that fit like grains of salt into every open space. In healthy enamel the crystals are separated by a thin, watery film between the crystals—the thinner this layer, the healthier the enamel will be, and the more your tooth will sparkle and shine. The strength and density of enamel fluctuates constantly, depending on how tightly the enamel crystals are packed within this lattice, as well as on the quality of the crystals themselves.

Inside enamel's lattice structure, these crystals are arranged in a complex but consistent manner. Most enamel crystals lie adjacent to one another, in an alignment that creates solid tube-shaped structures known as *enamel rods*. These crystalline rods travel in parallel and stretch the full thickness of the enamel, from the inside to outside of each tooth's enamel coating. Between these rods are contrasting areas that are packed with crystals arranged in a different and more curved fashion. These curves can appear haphazard, but they are, in fact, highly organized into a crisscrossed and interlocking configuration that offers exceptional strength to this thin enamel layer on the outside of your teeth. At a high microscopic resolution, it is possible to see that the structure of human enamel is consistent and that every tooth is similarly organized with these complex and intricate patterns.

One of the more surprising facts about enamel is that it is the hardest substance in the human body—harder even than *bone*. The hardness of enamel ranks "5" on the Moh's scale, a form of established measurement that serves to classify naturally occurring minerals into a ranked list where diamonds land at the top with a rating of "10." Moh's measurements tell us about the resistance of minerals to being scratched in any way—the hardness of a human fingernail or the mineral gold, for example, would produce a Moh's rating of less than "2.5." The measurement of "5" for enamel further indicates that healthy tooth enamel is less likely to be scratched than the metals of steel or iron, which have a lower Moh's number of "4.5." Enamel that has lost its hardness through exposure to acidity may, however, become softer than a fingernail and quite easily worn and scratched by many products—resulting in enamel wear, known as *abrasion*.

Enamel's unexpected strength stems partly from its mineral content, but also from the incredibly complex arrangement of the individual enamel crystals and from the way they adhere to one another. Enamel's microhardness can also be measured using what is called a Knoop Hardness Test (KHT), which determines the resilience of enamel by pressing into it with a diamond point. As a result, a Knoop Hardness Number (KHN) shows enamel's overall hardness as a measured range of "343 to 370," whereas the inside dentin of a tooth has a KHN of "68"—and this helps explain why dentin is so much more easily abraded or damaged than enamel.

This type of damage occurs—for example—when there is a "caving in" of the enamel shell of a tooth (as a cavity forms) and this exposes dentin to the mouth's environment, or when there is a loss of gum protection (because of gum disease), which allows softer dentin to be in contact with the mouth's environment and in real danger because it is *no longer* covered by strong tooth enamel or protected by normal gum tissues.

We have already discussed enamel and have explored its physical structure, but let's define it even more sharply at this point. Technically speaking, enamel is composed of natural *hydroxyapatite crystals*, and *hydroxyapatite* is a compound formed from the binding of calcium and phosphate—two minerals that occur at high levels in the spit that our mouths produce on a constant basis (and which is referred to in dentistry as our *saliva*). The acidity of liquids can easily be measured on a specific level of acidity, or *pH scale*. These measurements range from the numbers 0 to 14, where a neutral liquid is assigned a pH of "7." The saliva in our mouth can vary greatly in acidity. When it is flowing naturally, the pH measurement can fluctuate between pH "5" and "7.4," depending on many individual factors.

We find in all cases, however, that when saliva is stimulated to flow more rapidly (and we will discuss how this can occur later in this book), this stimulation immediately increases its pH to several numbers higher than its normal (or *resting*) pH level. When we measure minerals in saliva, we find that the less minerals the saliva carries, the lower its pH number. The higher the pH of saliva, the more minerals it will hold.

A healthy saliva measured at a pH of around "7.4" will, in fact, hold more minerals than expected. This is known as *super-saturation*—and as you can imagine, holding more minerals in solution is not a stable situation, so this so-called *metastable* state leaves saliva ready to change back to a more balanced state. This happens when saliva releases some of these excess minerals and deposits them on teeth. This is an amazing benefit for teeth, but specifically for the tooth's enamel shell covering. At a mouth pH level of "7.4," minerals will therefore move on automatically from our saliva and into any defects in the enamel surface with which it makes contact.

These minerals then diffuse and seep from the outside surface and into the enamel latticework, provided that our saliva is not diluted, thinned, or changed in any way. Here the minerals will either combine with existing crystals to expand their size, or they will seed new crystals to replace lost ones. The strength of enamel increases as the integrity of the structure develops, and as more and more minerals enter the lattice. As hydroxyapatite crystals from saliva fill all the open spaces, the tooth's enamel crystals become densely packed and thus create the solid, smooth enamel found in a healthy mouth. The physical structure of enamel unites high strength with extreme toughness, qualities that are not easily mimicked by synthetic materials.

Tooth enamel must withstand upwards of a million bites over a lifetime—bites that are created as the jaws clamp together, and which can produce a force equal to 224 pounds of pressure on the top of the tooth surfaces. Every molar tooth therefore needs to be strong enough to withstand high intermittent pressure without damage, if it is to offer sustained protection to the tooth's soft and valuable interior.

Not only is our tooth enamel strong, but it is also uniquely *personal*. In fact, it has been discovered in recent years that every person has a distinct pattern of enamel crystal design. Enamel crystals are grouped together to form enamel rods, and these radiate in a three-dimensional arch around the tooth's surface, curving in all directions. The rod structure gives our teeth extraordinary strength, and their design pattern recalls the construction systems used to generate passive strength in the building of cathedral arches. A *voussoir arch* is a building method where a central voussoir, or *keystone*, is used to supply critical arch strength. In a tooth, crystalline keystones do not work two-dimensionally but rather in a *three*-dimensional way.

Enamel design thus supports downward pressure by effectively forcing the enamel crystals together by compression, rather than apart. Here we see the way enamel derives its strength from its microscopic organization, and how forces are dissipated and released by the rods and crystals—scattering and radiating the forces through, and *over*, the entire tooth structure. So, when a dental drill cuts away the keystone crystals of enamel, the overall strength of the tooth is immediately compromised—and no filling will exactly repair or replace its original design.

The cutting of tooth enamel means it can no longer rely on its microscopic structure to dissipate the forces created by biting and chewing. The result is that these forces travel instead through the filling until they reach its base. Here they will spread sideways, shooting in a straight line toward the widest part of the tooth. This is how surface cracks can develop and become a vulnerable entry space for bacteria on the side surface of a tooth. If cavity bacteria floating in saliva gain access to a microscopic gap or crack, they can penetrate deep into the tooth and create a decay problem that is known as an *interproximal cavity*. Interproximal cavities often occur on several teeth simultaneously and are usually a secondary problem, discovered just a few years after one or two small central fillings or sealants have been placed on the top biting surface of a tooth.

Teeth offer us a varied collection of grinding and slicing surfaces that allow us to bite into and chew up every imaginable kind of food. The flatter molar teeth at the back of the mouth are useful for mashing or grinding food, while our front teeth efficiently incise or bite things. A tooth's vulnerability to damage is not related to its function, but its shape is most often the underlying reason why certain teeth are more vulnerable to fracture, erosion, or cavities. For example, the enamel in the center of a molar tooth is indented with deep grooves and, at their base, the enamel is thinner and more vulnerable to the attack of decay-causing bacteria than the thick smooth enamel covering the surface of a front *incisor*, or of a corner *canine* tooth.

Enamel may be strong, but it is not indestructible—as anyone who has had a cavity knows. When enamel crystals are weakened by acidity, small pieces of enamel can quite easily be shed or break off around the neck of a tooth, where the enamel crystals are shorter and have less strength as they are angled away from the biting surface. This is how channels of lost enamel can arise on the sides of teeth, creating a problem known as *enamel erosion*. The damage usually affects several teeth at the same time, most often on the outside surfaces of upper or lower molars.

Dentists are trained to recognize which teeth are more easily damaged and therefore know where to look for the first signs of erosion or decay—problems that occur in certain areas of specific teeth in a relatively predictable sequence. This explains why dentists learn so much about tooth anatomy and it can assist them in their daily task of inspecting tooth surfaces, so they know where to look for cracks; dark spots of decay; the gray hue of a dead tooth; or the brown lines that can signal a breach in the tooth's integrity.

Do *not* let the fact that some teeth are vulnerable to decay fool you, though. Enamel has the power to heal itself under the right conditions, and it is also incredibly durable. In 2022, a 1.8-million-year-old human tooth was discovered near Tbilisi, the capital of the East European nation of Georgia near the Mtkvari River on the Eastern end of the Black Sea. To date, this is the most ancient tooth ever discovered. Furthermore, in 2015 scientists in southern China discovered forty-seven human teeth that have since been dated back to the prehistoric year of 77000 BCE. Some of these ancient teeth may have a few erosion marks on their surface, but their overall condition is spectacular after so many thousands of years, and without any sign of cavities.

Yet even though teeth are strong enough to survive long after the body has disintegrated, it is easy for us to unknowingly create situations that overwhelm their defenses and deactivate the mouth's repair systems. Tooth enamel is vulnerable to acidic attack and therefore to the development of tooth weakness and the acid-promoted disease that results in all kinds of tooth damage and cavities. The saliva in our mouth, when it is healthy, provides everything a tooth needs to repair enamel, and the dentin layer (inside this enamel shell) is home to cells that can sense danger, and which even have an ability to secrete a cement-like barrier that can slowly block off incoming damage or disease. (Saliva will be discussed in greater detail in Chapter Three.) And so, with much of our oral health reliant on the body's ability to provide dependable protection, it is crucial that our lifestyle choices not get in the way of what nature has already given us.

Dentistry Endgame—*Now* What?

The problem for our body and mouth is that often the body's natural repair systems are confronted with a barrage of assaults from the phenomena of the modern age—and this includes everything from damage caused by whitening procedures, a loss of minerals from careless daily habits, or those hidden danger signals that are being muffled by desensitizing oral care products—or simply ignored because we don't know what to do. There are so many things that abuse or disable the body's regeneration system, and we court danger whenever we flood our mouths with dangerous acidity from soft drinks and fast foods; take medications that decrease our saliva flow; ingest a steady diet of sugary and high carbohydrate foods; or live with so much continual stress that it depletes our saliva of essential minerals.

In addition, many people live and interact in crowded communities, at least for a part of their lives—at high school, at college, during hospital stays, or later in life at assisted living centers. In these situations, our mouths can be exposed more prevalently to waves of directly transmissible oral and tooth infection, which can come from others living in these communities or from hugging and kissing with family and friends. Infection by cavity-forming plaque bacteria can easily wreck teeth, sometimes so rapidly that a baby tooth can become decayed almost before it has had time to grow and line up in the mouth. Tooth damage and disease is not the result of faulty natural tooth design. Instead, it more frequently results from an imbalance created by habits of constant eating and drinking and a lack of understanding about how to effectively support the incredible yet *invisible* mouth defense systems that have the power to protect and restore our teeth and gums.

White Fangs?

A tooth's outer enamel crystals are colorless and transparent, akin to a clear glass window. However, when these enamel crystals come together to form enamel, they start to refract and reflect light in a way that gives teeth their white appearance. This visual illusion is orchestrated by a watery layer surrounding each crystal, and it is the consistency of this liquid that alters the trajectory of light. In healthy enamel, the result is a sparkling, brilliant tooth, reminiscent of a diamond that is in fact a clear, translucent crystal but appears to the eye as a radiant, white gem. Unfortunately, the aim of many "tooth-whitening" products is to disrupt this delicate water balance between the enamel crystals, replacing the water with air or other substances that alter light's interaction with our tooth enamel. This is how artificial whitening products change the color of teeth and why they often give them an unnatural, uniform, and often chalky, ultra-white hue.

While these alterations may produce the desired illusion, it is crucial to recognize that such tricks contribute nothing to oral health. For anyone who wants to naturally whiten their teeth, the key is to help your teeth become fully mineralized. This means correct care, which includes carefully avoiding prolonged periods of acidity, damage from products that strip teeth of their natural protection, and avoidance of sensitive or so-called "mineralizing" toothpastes that usually create a barrier over the enamel surface, which can potentially obstruct or prevent this natural process of enamel mineralization.

Other tooth-color enhancing products may be potentially harmful because they etch, scrub, or *bleach* the tooth surface. Many individuals mistakenly believe that the more we polish our teeth, the brighter they will be, but this too is untrue. Delicate crystals can be eroded by abrasive oral care products, and acidity will dissolve away minerals, leaving a tooth vulnerable to wear, changes of color, fractures, sensitivity, and infection. The apparent increase in demand for bite plates and night guards may have nothing to do with an increase in tooth grinding, but rather an epidemic of weakened tooth enamel caused by modern snacking habits, tooth whitening, and constant sipping of sparkling water, energy and sports drinks, gummy candies and vitamins, sugary chews, and supplements—all of which may contain enough citric acid to dissolve tooth enamel.

The natural renewal of enamel can only occur under reasonable circumstances and, once this level of abuse tolerance has been breached, not only will it become harder to restore lost minerals, but there is also some danger that the vulnerable interior of the tooth will become sensitive to temperature changes in the mouth and infections caused by intruding plaque bacteria. The tooth's core pulp, which houses live cells and nerves, desperately needs to be protected by healthy enamel. Inflammation or infection of these interior tissues can cause swelling to occur inside the confined pulp space in the center of the tooth, and this can lead to an increase in pressure that may be sufficient to crush the tooth's nerves, limit its blood supply, and literally kill the tooth. Many artificial whitening products breach the enamel layer with strong acids so that protein-altering compounds can change the color of the tooth's interior dentin. Pulp inflammation has been observed—sometimes lasting for weeks—after this kind of tooth-bleaching procedure. Tooth death may not be evident for ten to fifteen years after the initial irritation, noticeable as a little tooth sensitivity or pulp discomfort, but which eventually and slowly progresses to tooth death.

It has often been said that one must suffer to be beautiful, but this extreme kind of product-inflicted damage to our teeth is ridiculous—and it needs to be *stopped*.

CONCLUSION

In this chapter, we have looked closely at what can be found in the human mouth—elements both visible, like teeth and gums, and *invisible*, which is practically everything else. We also looked into some of the reasons why so many of us dread going to the dentist, and how improvement to our daily home maintenance can make a difference to our dental visits and help us to conquer that fear. Lastly, we took a deep dive into the key systems of repair that occur in our mouths every day—and *why* so many people end up on a downward slide toward increasingly frequent dental appointments, and *bills*, by taking for granted the remarkable world of biology and interwoven chemistry that exists to heal our mouths . . . if we would only tend to it.

The teeth that we are able to *see* in our mouths live in a naturally occurring *partnership* with all the invisible life and liquid chemistry that surrounds them—all day, and all through the night. This delicate interplay continues to fill me as a dental professional with wonder and awe—particularly as tooth cells, nerves, and regenerative enamel crystals all work together in seemingly magical ways. My hope is that this beautiful picture of mouth harmony, with all its natural splendor, will help everyone begin to appreciate why their teeth are so precious and valuable; why careless or inappropriate home care is more than just a mistake; and why harmful, or *unnecessary*, dental treatments should never be accepted as inevitable or—worse yet—that cavities and gum disease typify a kind of collectively uncontrollable, or progressively destructive, fate. And as we move into the next chapters, this is a good time for a reminder that we have more control over our mouth health than we may think—if we can embrace and *appreciate* the power of prevention.

3

$\mathcal{S}$aliva's Got a Secret—
And It's Time to Spit It Out

Getting well is easy, it is getting sick
that takes years of constant, dedicated hard work.
—DR. RICHARD SCHULZE

We all know what *spit* is—but what, some might ask, is *saliva*? It turns out that they are the same thing—the spit in our mouth is a naturally occurring secretion officially called *saliva*. An adequate flow of this unique substance is essential for oral health, and the protection it offers is the result of the many component ingredients that work together to keep our mouth in perfect harmony. If this flow of saliva is reduced for any reason, or its composition is changed and becomes *less* protective, then tooth damage and disease are likely to occur in the mouth.

This is frequently the starting point for nearly *all* cavities and gum disease. When it comes down to it, saliva remains one of our strongest *secret* weapons in our struggle to maintain optimal balance in our mouth. Consider the following idea:

Our mouth health is a canvas.

Our teeth are works of art.

And our saliva can be seen as a renewable
and remarkable coat of protective paint.

Saliva plays many important roles when it comes to keeping things healthy in our mouths. When this protection works in synergy, it keeps our mouth healthy—but often we are unaware of saliva's benefits and simply believe that we are *lucky* benefactors of effortless oral health. It may be a stroke of luck for you, but in reality, it is another example of the way our body has power to control disease and create a positive health balance.

Saliva is *also* a lubricant that moistens the mouth and aids us when we swallow food. It keeps the lining of the mouth and teeth adequately hydrated and protected from mechanical damage that often occurs as we chew and consume foods of different textures. Saliva is such a helpful ally to us when it comes to our digestion. It serves to dissolve tasty particles from foods, which allows us to experience a vast assemblage of culinary flavors through the taste buds on our tongue. This, of course, makes eating that much more enjoyable and safer for our total body health—and we have saliva to thank for it.

Certain immune proteins in saliva play an antimicrobial role and help to clear bacteria from the mouth, while other proteins exert a healing effect on gum and mouth tissues. Over 300 kinds of proteins have been identified in saliva, and potentially more interactions and benefits will be discovered as salivary research expands in the future. Enzymes in saliva initiate important digestive processes in the mouth, especially the breakdown of carbohydrates, which are separated into more digestible sugars before being swallowed.

Recent work has focused on genetic markers discovered in saliva, which can be used to diagnose dysfunction and disease in other parts of the body. This kind of testing may one day put dentists in a more preventive health care role, where they potentially become primary providers for identification—through salivary testing—of all manner of important information about a patient's overall health, even incorporating breath technology where volatile organic compounds in breath become signals called *biomarkers* that alert us to early cancer, bacterial imbalances, and diseased organs.

Saliva has an ever-changing composition, and the total mix of its ingredients—at any given moment in time—is called *whole saliva*.

This liquid will usually contain a high number of *electrolytes* (electrically charged natural minerals found in one's blood and other bodily fluids) along with immune cells and a varied range of proteins, in proportions that are constantly changing. Saliva is squeezed out from two major glands that are found on each side of the jawbone—one in each cheek of the face, and one at the back of the nose. Each gland generates, modifies, and paces the secretion of saliva's various elements, which are then pumped automatically along ducts that travel from these glands and into the mouth, with openings under our tongue and on the inside of our cheek. These salivary variations are influenced by hormones (and the resultant emotions that we experience), circulation, digestive health, and biologic commands that originate from our nervous system.

This changing composition and flow rate has other influencing factors, including messaging from the nerves that connect to our eyes and to our sense of smell. This means the rate saliva flows into our mouth is variable, and these differences are layered over a flow speed that automatically fluctuates with a repetitive 24-hour cycle, every day and night, a variation that we first identified in Chapter One as a *Circadian rhythm*. These alterations in saliva quality are important because the varying chemistry creates either a positive influence on our mouth, or it can be a hindrance to our oral health efforts.

The overall quality of our saliva naturally ebbs and flows almost every hour of every day. In the morning hours, saliva can be somewhat more acidic—but after midday, most people find that their saliva is a higher pH (less acidic) and more healing. Since the health of saliva is also quickly reflected by our diet, noontime is perhaps the ideal time for saliva-promoting foods like salads and greens, that can enhance this naturally healing afternoon saliva flow.

The main concern is to stop snacking and sipping during the time when you have quality saliva in your mouth. Another way to benefit from saliva is to stimulate a flow with some xylitol, and then do not eat or drink for one or more hours afterward to allow this healing saliva adequate time to mineralize your teeth and heal your gums. (Look ahead in Part Two of this book for more details on xylitol.)

The most difficult time for mouth health is while we are sleeping at night. This is because saliva's Circadian rhythm reduces saliva flow during the night, and it is more acidic in the hours after midnight—when we are sleeping. This acidity and reduced flow can leave our teeth and mouth dry and unprotected. If a dry mouth and lack of saliva is a bother to you at night, start by considering the value of rest and relaxation—which have a beneficial effect on saliva flow—especially before sleeping at night. This lack of help from saliva during the night also makes it important to use a well-selected oral care routine prior to sleeping. (In Part Two we will discuss in further detail my Complete Mouth Care System™, which helps to keep teeth safe during this difficult time in the night.)

ACIDIC SALIVA

For oral health we want our saliva to be perfect, pristine, and the carrier of minerals and immune cells into our mouth. Sometimes, unfortunately, you may find that your mouth's saliva is acidic, and then, no matter how well you brush and floss, you will be at a higher risk for cavities and tooth decay. We can test the acidity of our saliva by allowing the liquid in our mouth to pool on the tip of our tongue, and then spit this into a spoon. We can dip the end of an absorbent paper strip (called *litmus paper*) into this spat-out sample, and the special dyes in litmus paper will change color to illustrate the acidity of the sample (which, as defined earlier in this book, is called our saliva's *pH*).

The measuring scale for pH levels is between zero and fourteen, so that a pH of 7 would indicate a non-acidic or *neutral state*. If this pH test is taken with normally flowing saliva in your mouth (which is called *resting saliva*), and if the result is neutral or slightly alkaline (around a pH of 7.4), then this would be considered a healthy result. At a pH of around 7.4, saliva has a composition that will be able to defend the integrity of your gums and the skin of your mouth (known as the *oral epithelium*). It will also be able to transport sufficient minerals for the maintenance, health, and strength of one's teeth.

The "It" of Spit When You Eat

As mentioned, saliva pH is rarely constant, and it can change for many reasons. Some of the most dramatic changes in saliva's pH occur when we eat or drink. Many foods reduce our mouth to a low pH of around 5 or 6, and some foods and drinks can even cause the mouth pH level to dip between 2 and 4. Whenever the mouth's acidity level falls below 6, every tooth surface is at risk for mineral loss. Harmful plaque bacteria also gain momentum in acidic mouth conditions and will use this pH to their benefit and form thick plaque on tooth surfaces, where multiplying bacteria can damage our teeth and gums.

There is a direct mixing of drinks with our saliva as we sip and consume them. The beverage entering our mouth immediately dilutes the consistency of normal saliva, and the two different liquids quickly intermingle to create a pH that is approximately an *average* between their different pH values. While we eat meals, soluble ingredients from food dissolve in saliva. These saliva/food and saliva/drink mixtures then circulate everywhere in our mouth—they touch every tooth surface, and enter every groove, pit, or gap in and between teeth, fillings, or crowns, flowing between teeth—even teeth that appear very tight and crowded.

This means that all meals, snacks, and drinks—even a sip of water—will change the composition of our saliva and potentially disable its healing quality. Any drop in the mouth's pH levels will also pull minerals *from* tooth surfaces. As a result, any lingering or prolonged periods of acidity will likely promote negative changes in the health of our tooth enamel and encourage less beneficial bacteria to populate our mouth.

Alas, this is why frequent eating, snacking, and especially the sipping of beverages will stress teeth, gums, and our overall mouth health. Especially damaging are any foods and drinks that contain carbohydrates, sugars, strong acids (like *phosphoric* or *citric acid*, which are found in many flavored waters and sodas), or even a consistent consumption of carbonated sparkling drinks—which, of course, *also* can make the mouth highly acidic. Remember that story you heard once about how soda drinks can peel the paint off an automobile? Just think about what those same destructive liquids are doing to the inside of your mouth!

Saliva and the Sugar Cycle

In the mouth, it is specific plaque- and cavity-forming bacteria that metabolize sugars from our diet. When we consume any sugar-containing or carbohydrate-rich foods, these sugars they contain will dissolve in saliva and be transported around the mouth to feed these harmful bacteria. This situation occurs almost instantly as the food enters the mouth, which does not give anyone time to run and clean their teeth to stop the interaction. The sugar can nourish plaque bacteria, especially any located on the surface of teeth, which will be able to use this energy to multiply and grow thicker and more hazardous to your teeth and gums. The byproduct of growing plaque is an acidic liquid, which seeps through the plaque mass to damage teeth but also to mix with saliva and create even more acidic mouth conditions—which then favor even *more* plaque growth.

Constant snacking, especially with sugary or carbohydrate-rich foods or the sipping of any sugary or acidic drinks, causes plaque to grow into a thick mass on teeth. This unhealthy cycle is the main cause of cavities, filling deterioration, and the first stage of gum disease that is called *gingivitis*.

There remains a misconception in our culture that sugar and sweets are to blame for tooth decay—and certainly sugars are a part of this unhealthy saliva sugar cycle. Make no mistake: It is possible to give up the consumption of all sugary and carbohydrate foods and, if you carefully brush and floss, be able to improve and maybe control *some* dental problems. If, however, your mouth is acidic, then sugar control, even with excellent brushing and flossing, will not offer sufficient protection.

Your acidic saliva will continue to create tooth-damaging and plaque-forming conditions in your mouth—despite your oral health efforts and sugar-restrictive diet. Conversely, it is not necessary to insist on a completely sugar- and carbohydrate-deprived diet for oral health. If you do not like the idea of dietary restrictions, be encouraged because mouth health can be controlled by the timing and frequency of your grazing, snacks, sweets, meals, drinks, gummies, protein bars, chewable vitamins, and other fun foods that are known to cause tooth decay. In fact, if we want to point a finger of judgment at all the things that damage oral health, then we should also direct this to every sip of water or liquid (sugary or not) that changes the composition of saliva, as diluted or thin saliva can play its own deleterious role.

Now don't panic—and please don't think that you can never eat or drink anything again. Quite the opposite, in fact. The good news is that you have almost total flexibility about your food choices at every meal and snack, without limitations or even sugar restrictions. All we need to do is corral our eating or drinking sessions into a reasonable number of times each day—and I suggest to clients that this should be a daily total of five (5) to six (6) meals/snacks/drinks, each of 15 to 60 minutes' duration. One thing to realize here is that the longer you take to consume meals, snacks, and drinks, the more potential there is for tooth damage to occur. With this approach there is no longer any list of taboo foods or drinks, since nothing you eat will cause damage if you end your meals with a tooth-protective food. This way of eating will allow you to enjoy the foods you wish—provided that you know *how* and *when* to eat and drink and still ensure the safety of your oral health.

SWEET SALIVA

As we eat foods, the particles of food are crushed by our teeth and then mix into our mouth's saliva. Dissolved in saliva these food particles are carried through our mouth, mixed together with all our mouth liquids. Any sugars from food dissolves instantly, but carbo-hydrates are also quickly broken down into smaller particle sugars by enzymes in saliva. This means that any sugars create a sweet solution of saliva that flows everywhere in your mouth, feeding all the sugar-loving, acid-producing, plaque-forming bacteria lodged in every nook and cranny of your teeth—and even the bacteria floating in saliva and on the skin of your mouth and throat—in places that cannot be cleaned by either brushing or flossing.

This explains why people who meticulously clean their teeth can still wind up with cavities and gum disease because of their eating habits and patterns. It also explains why trying to clean your teeth after a meal is ineffective to stop this kind of damage, which occurs almost instantaneously—seconds after a nibble on that sugary carbohydrate or acidic food. The time interval between the act of eating food or sipping a drink and the resultant pH change is immediate, making it impossible to "brush your teeth" and prevent this damage, no matter what you were told as a child.

The acidity caused each time we eat can cause a pH drop in the mouth that will continue for up to an hour. This acidic environment can promote harmful bacteria and may dissolve minerals from the enamel of your teeth. Eating multiple times each day simply adds multiple hours of extended acidic damage. This may sound depressing but read on because you can easily limit this post-meal period of acidity and turn acidic saliva back into a naturally occurring *tooth-healing* saliva. This needs to happen each time after we eat or drink, so that we can replace any lost minerals and repair any "demineralization" damage.

HOW TO IMPROVE SALIVA HEALTH

It should by now be obvious that our saliva can be impacted directly by almost *anything* we put into our mouths. For instance, smoking and vaping are damaging habits that dramatically affect the composition and flow of saliva—and this, of course, will serve to dry the mouth and reduce or eliminate saliva's health benefits. Many familiar medications can *also* create dry mouth problems and, in this way, suddenly increase someone's risk *for* cavities and gum disease.

So, now let's look together at the actual health of saliva as it enters your mouth. Poor-quality saliva can be the outcome of a bad diet. However, it can also be a silent symptom of:

- Our digestive health;

- Inadequate rest and sleep;

- Insufficient exercise;

- Medication side effects;

- The result of stress or hormonal imbalances (especially during pregnancy, menopause, and in later life); or

- A consequence of open-mouth breathing, sinus infections, allergies, and possibly the result of wearing dental braces and retainers (which impedes saliva flow).

Our saliva provides transportation and dietary support to the large assortment of bacteria that live in our mouths. Approximately twenty percent (20%) of the mouth's bacterial community float freely in this liquid and travel wherever saliva travels, in and out of teeth, and down the throat and into the digestive tract. The majority of mouth bacteria, however, are also nurtured by saliva, but they do *not* float in the mouth liquids. Instead, this eighty percent (80%) portion of the mouth's bacteria is wrapped in protein strands and covers all the surfaces of our mouth, teeth, and gums. This film of bacteria woven in a web of proteins is called *oral biofilm*, and its health is influenced directly by the quality and features of our mouth's saliva.

For example, healthy biofilm is damaged if it loses moisture for an extended period. When saliva dries up or does not coat tooth surfaces adequately, or if saliva is unable to keep the gums moist, this is when the protective oral biofilm shrinks, and this can expose tooth and gum surfaces to harmful bacteria—and a risk of infection. How we breathe, our stress levels, and even hormonal shifts can cause saliva to flow less fluidly, become too dilute, or ineffective—all factors that will damage the health of our mouth biofilm.

So how can you fight back and manage the health of your saliva, so that you can support the health of your biofilm—the film that protects our teeth and gums from damage and disease? This question is especially important if you are taking medications that dry your mouth or if you have allergies that make you breathe more through your mouth.

The first place to look is at the foods you are eating regularly. Certain foods will benefit the biofilm directly—fruits like raspberries and blackberries—which themselves contain the natural sugar xylitol, also shown to have protective effects within the mouth. Other studies show how vegetables normally served in salads—lettuce, cucumber, celery, and beets, in particular—support the production of an altogether healthier alkaline mouth environment, which over time will impact the health of your teeth and gums. Salty foods, cheeses, and oily foods (like avocado) are also on the list of foods that are called *tooth-protective* because they are helpful, not harmful, and because they can help generate and maintain a healthy saliva flow.

It may seem discouraging to think that everything we consume can damage our teeth and gums. You may feel frustrated to know that even water can thin and dilute the saliva, thus making it impotent when it comes to healing teeth. Consider, for example, that the commercially available Fiji and Evian waters each have a pH of 7.4 (equivalent to the exact pH of healthy saliva), but although they do not add any acidity into the mouth, these waters will dilute and thin saliva. And so, although they are not in themselves harmful to teeth, they are not as helpful as saliva.

Now, let's quickly agree that drinking water is a *healthy habit*. What we need to do is drink water without allowing it to dilute our valuable saliva. So, what is the answer? The solution is to generally drink either before, during, or after mealtimes—and less during intervals between meals. If you do not want to drink at meals, then you can just set aside some other "water snack" times during each day when you drink more than a sip or two at a time. In recent years, more health practitioners have begun to recommend that people should limit snacks and create boundaries for their eating routines, so this advice should fit into that approach—keeping our food and drinks within a schedule, as opposed to one that is continuous and never-ending each day from morning until night.

My career began working in a dental office that recommended

the adding of tooth-protective foods to the end of meals—for their protective effect. There are various of these food options (as we have discussed), and some people will want to explore these—but if you have a busy life and need a convenient and arguably ultimate tooth-protective food, let me suggest *xylitol*. Little mints and chewing gum sweetened with xylitol are amazing tooth-protective foods and are particularly helpful for people with a dry mouth or anyone experiencing chronic dental or gum problems. (You can read more about xylitol in Part Two.)

WHAT DOES "HPV" HAVE TO DO WITH ORAL HEALTH?

The eighty percent (80%) of mouth bacteria that do not float around in saliva are the bacteria we are going to consider next. This is because they are the most ignored and least understood, and they create the special biofilm that exists over the entire surface of the mouth. When the mouth is healthy, this translucent film stands as our best ally to manage the onslaught of "intruder" bacteria that come into our mouths from the world around us.

The integrity of healthy oral biofilm can help reject intruder bacteria traveling in saliva droplets that are shared when we talk and interact with one another. Healthy biofilm can work as an almost-bulletproof shield against other assaults that can cause damage to our teeth and gums. Healthy biofilm's bacterial communities live as a communicating unit within its mesh-like structure, with a wide variety of healthy bacteria that are able to coexist with each other and perform as if in unison—like a well-organized army—exhibiting characteristics that are more potent and defensive than any individual bacteria could muster if it were floating individually in saliva liquids. Our biofilm protection covers our teeth, gums, and the skin inside our mouth, defending these surfaces from physical trauma that could otherwise cause ulceration and from infections by fungi, intruder viruses, or bacteria that could otherwise cause conditions such as the often-experienced fungal mouth infections known as *candida, lichen planus,* and *thrush.*

If our biofilm protection dries out (because saliva flow is slow or stopped), then this can leave the mouth more vulnerable to ulcers, tooth enamel erosion, cavities, and gum infection. Damage from wrong oral care by artificial whitening products, hydrogen peroxide, or baking soda, for example, or from chemo- or radiation therapy, and even from deep dental cleanings, can strip away our mouth's protective biofilm and open the door for problems of every kind, even the possibility—in some specific situations—of infection by the *Human Papilloma Virus* (HPV).

The Viral—and *Bacterial*—Dance of Love

The Human Papilloma Virus (HPV) is a sexually transmitted virus, and it is one of the most common sexually transmitted infections today in the United States. HPV is transferred through skin-to-skin contact and by oral sex, and HPV has the potential to raise someone's risk for cancer in areas of the mouth and throat.

HPV is the leading cause of oropharyngeal cancers today, primarily discovered in the tonsils, base of the tongue, throat, or at the front of the mouth. The Centers for Disease Control note that 10% of men and 3.6% of women test positive for oral HPV, and that the percentages increase with age. HPV may be more of a danger if the mouth's protective biofilm has been damaged or stripped away.

As the statistics show, more males than females develop HPV-associated oral cancers, and to explain this, a study by Gillison suggests females often become infected by HPV early in their sexual life, but rapidly develop a systemic antibody, which offers a full-body protection throughout life. Protection takes longer to develop in males, and it may require multiple exposures to HPV for a male to generate his immune response. This may be part of the reason why oral cancer in men is increasing in the age range 35–55, and why men are more at risk for oral cancer than women by a ratio of 4 to 1.

Fear of virus transmission can be alarming, as witnessed during the initial COVID-19 epidemic of 2020–2021. It is important to remember that the human body is beautifully equipped to resist invasion from intruder bacteria, provided that your defense systems are healthy and functioning. Problems occur when these protective systems are breached or overwhelmed, in what is commonly referred to as "perfect storm" situations.

Despite the resilience of oral biofilm, many medications, antibiotics, and even routine daily habits can damage this barrier—creating a portal for viral or bacterial infection to enter the mouth from one partner to the other. A defensive biofilm is found everywhere inside our nose, sinuses, and lungs—and it is useful to know that small amounts of xylitol (see Part Two) can help keep our mouth and nasal biofilms healthier.

HPV is a widespread viral infection, and at least one person develops an oral HPV infection in America every 20 minutes—with 26 million Americans currently infected by the HPV virus, according to the National Health And Nutrition Examination Survey (NHANES), which is a nationally representative study that has assessed the overall health of children and adults in the United States since 1999. This certainly *sounds* alarming—but before you rush to be tested, let's consider the other side of the equation.

There are over 200 strains of HPV, and the commonly used Polymerase Chain Reaction (PCR) test developed in 1983 is not only prone to error, but we know that only one percent (1%) of individuals testing HPV-positive will be at risk of this infection cascading into cancer (and this may actually occur many decades after the original infection).

HPV-16 is the primary cause of oral cancer today, surpassing tobacco and alcohol, but it appears that tobacco and excessive alcohol will increase this risk. Other more positive studies show drinking twenty-four (24) ounces of coffee per day (about 3–4 cups) can offer up to fifty percent (50%) protection from oral cancer. Fruits, vegetables, and green tea are other foods that can support our immune system and be protective and helpful.

The connection between intimacy and shared bacteria and viruses is a developing science—and it does appear that the greater the number of sexual partners, the more likely a person is to contract an HPV infection, and this applies as equally true for oral sex. PCR salivary testing continues to be a primary way to determine HPV levels and search specifically for HPV-16, the virus associated with throat, cervical, anal, and penile cancers. Most people—even those with the 16, high-risk version of HPV—do not develop cancer, and often do not show symptoms. HPV also goes into long periods of dormancy over decades, which explains why PCR testing is being questioned by experts in this field, and why it may be preferable to have a visual oral cancer screening with an oral surgeon before having any additional PCR testing as necessary.

Risks from Transmission

As humans, we are always at significant risk from bacterial transmission during skin-to-skin contact, and this is especially true between intimate partners. As previously mentioned, our mouth and nose are home to hundreds of different kinds of bacteria, most of which are healthy and helpful, and the biofilm covering our mouth and nose offers a defense against itinerant or intruder bacteria. Every part of the human skin covering the inside and outside of our bodies is host to its own specific and diverse bacterial community. Problems only occur when something upsets this normal balance and allows harm-causing bacteria to overgrow their normal levels and become dominant—often the result of changes caused by certain medications, a depleted immune response, or bacterial upset caused by antibiotic therapy.

The transfer of harmful bacteria can cause unexpected mouth problems in a partner, so this possibility will now be discussed while working to keep these concerns in perspective. There is substantial oral health risk for romantic partners to consider at any stage of life—particularly if someone is taking medications; is older or has a compromised immune system; or for anyone after a course of antibiotics.

There is always potential, however, for harmful plaque or *periodontal* (gum disease) pathogens to transfer in droplets of saliva during any intimate contact, and even when talking or simply living in a shared physical space. Typically, partners who are together for years will experience this transfer—and if they are able to maintain oral health, can potentially reap the benefits from a wider diversity of bacteria in their biofilm.

In 1970, we learned from dental studies that plaque bacteria from a mother's mouth easily populates the teeth of her baby—and this transfer influences the child's oral health for life. Sharing chronic periodontal gum disease bacteria can be very problematic for partners, because the infection they cause is below the gums and may not cause any visible or tangible symptoms. Periodontal disease involves a specific group of bacteria that multiply in low oxygen conditions as single cells in saliva and travel from the throat, mouth, and sinus in the liquids that circulate in these areas. They are present in the mouths of most adults and reach high levels in people who have chronic periodontal disease, sinus infections, and often in the airways of those with chronic breathing issues.

These harmful bacteria cannot be brushed or flossed from salivary liquids but flow wherever body liquids flow—even into our digestive tract. These are the bacteria that can cause serious damage to our gums if they lodge alongside a tooth inside a dark, low oxygen space called a *periodontal pocket*. These bacteria can infect the mouth of a partner if this partner has periodontal pockets, often causing deterioration in the partner's oral health both silently and rapidly.

The speed and severity of a transferred periodontal problem will depend on the recipient's immune system health; their absence or presence of periodontal pockets in their gums; their daily mouth care; and overall health and habits. The risk of transfer can occur whenever we live closely with *any* individual who has chronic gum disease, recurring sinus infections, or breathing problems. Those who engage in oral sex should also be aware that specific bacteria, most often recognized as contributors to periodontal disease, can transfer to or from the vagina of a partner.

Oral salivary testing is available to determine the pathogen levels in your mouth, but at present this new science seems to be creating as many questions as it provides answers. The specific bacteria that are implicated in this kind of transfer are: *porphyromonas, prevotella, peptostreptococcus*, and *fusobacterium* bacteria. *Porphyromonas gingivalis* (PG) and *Aggregatibacter actinomycetemcomitans* (AA) are two highly transmissible and aggressive periodontal pathogens, with the ability to breach the skin surface that allows them to both damage gum tissues and potentially invade the body to cause chronic inflammation around the heart, joints, brain, and gut. PG and AA pathogens may also shorten the gestation period for an unborn baby, which is how gum disease raises a pregnant woman's risk for pre-term birth.

Interestingly, a 2022 study in Malawi showed that two pieces of one hundred percent (100%) xylitol gum—one gram consumed before sleeping every night and the other after lunch—was able to significantly reduce this risk of pre-term birth. New studies are looking at changes in the periodontal pathogens with xylitol use in pregnant women, and perhaps we can hypothesize that xylitol may exert an effect on PG and AA levels in the mouth.

Kissing and sharing bathroom spaces appears to be major contributing factors for sharing periodontal bacteria in close quarters, and usually this requires contact for more than a day. The recipient of the periodontal pathogens floating into his or her mouth will only be vulnerable if they have periodontal pocketing, which is why being vigilant to eliminate any periodontal pocketing is so important for your overall health. People without this type of gum pocketing condition in their mouths have no suitable habitat for the multiplication of periodontal bacteria—and so they are relatively safe, as a result.

How to Keep Oral Biofilm Healthy

As we have by now firmly established, healthy oral biofilm is critical for the maintenance and defense of your mouth health. Healthy saliva supports the integrity of tooth enamel and also the health of oral biofilm. Sometimes during hormonal change and pregnancy, it can be almost impossible to control the acidity of saliva, and this is when teeth and gums need extra help.

If you are experiencing hormonal changes; are stressed, or pregnant; if you take medications that dry your mouth (allergy medications, blood pressure medication, and diuretics, for example); if you have had a course of radiation or chemotherapy; or if you have an autoimmune problem that has attacked your salivary glands, then you will need to understand the many ways we can directly assist our saliva to protect our mouth—and avoid the many problems that have too often been accepted as uncontrollable, age-related, or inherited. The variable least appreciated is the value obtained from the interaction of undiluted saliva with our mouth and teeth each day. We must consider this—especially for anyone at risk for problems—if we are to help maintain oral health for life.

Stimulated saliva is a perfect solution to counteract the loss of minerals from teeth that occurs in every mouth, every time we eat and drink. Those at higher risk because of a dry mouth or acidic saliva can use stimulated saliva as their personal rescue resource. Stimulated saliva has an exceptional load of minerals suspended in it, as it is emitted from the salivary glands. This kind of highly mineralized liquid is known by chemists as a *super-saturated solution*. In other words, minerals are virtually dripping out of saliva as they flow into the mouth, immediately ready to coat the surface of our teeth and mineralize, heal, and beautify them on contact.

In the end, there is no way we can brush, polish, or shine teeth as effectively as healthy saliva's daily interaction with our tooth enamel. Oral health problems will always occur when saliva is devoid of minerals, is frequently thinned by the liquids we sip, and when saliva flow is interrupted or reduced.

CONCLUSION

Your dentist can physically repair and clean your teeth, but he or she *cannot* make your saliva healthier. This is something we must do for ourselves. As we bring this chapter to a close, here is a review of the three most important things to consider for the support of your saliva health.

1. Saliva is a valuable and "secret"—or as-yet unrecognized—weapon in your oral health arsenal. Its underappreciated benefits can be compromised by careless eating and drinking habits. Try to reasonably control your daily eating and drinking sessions, ending each meal, if possible, with a tooth-protective food—followed by a period of *mouth resting* for at least an hour, and ideally longer.

2. Our entire body works as an interconnected unit, and saliva health demonstrates how impulses generated by stimuli from our eyes, nose, and even emotions can change the composition and texture of the saliva in our mouth. Take time before eating to rest and relax, or maybe at least a few seconds to observe and appreciate the food you are going to consume. Your saliva will thank you for this relaxing gesture and, in return, you may discover it delivers positive contributions to your teeth and overall health.

3. Healthy saliva helps maintain a delicate balance of *good* bacteria in our mouths. Mouth bacteria are associated with the first stages of digestion for certain foods, and many oral bacteria are swallowed in the saliva that moistens food. Healthy digestion encourages more nutrients to enter our blood and be transported around the body. Healthy digestion also nurtures our immune system, and supports the production of immune cells, proteins, and the antibodies that help us fight disease. Exercise circulates blood around our body and into the vascular salivary glands nestled in our face. In these glands there is a direct exchange of nutrients, immune cells, and proteins that go from the blood into the salivary fluids, which are then squeezed into the mouth. These nutrients, cells, and proteins are the essential components that help saliva maintain a healthy balance of good bacteria in the mouth, to aid in the digestion of food—and so, the salivary circle of health repeats.

   In the next chapter, we will take an in-depth look at white and silver amalgam fillings, flossing, and fluoridation—areas of oral care that have just about as many dentists who endorse them as dentists who *don't*.

4

$\mathcal{F}$lossing, Fillings, and Fluoridation— The Three "Fs" of Dentistry

I am lying—true or false?

—PARAPHRASE OF GREEK PHILOSOPHER EUBULIDES' "LIAR PARADOX" (*DATE UNKNOWN*)

So, we all know that we must clean our teeth, but how can we do that in a way that encourages superior oral health—and keeps dental problems at a minimum? Well, the American Dental Association (ADA) recommends that we brush and floss and have semi-annual dental cleanings. However, statistics continuously show—including those generated by the National Health and Nutrition Examination Survey (NHANES)—that ninety-six percent (96%) of Americans retire with cavities, extracted teeth, fillings, root canals, and gum disease—even dentists, who should be the "brush and floss" experts. Financial planners warn us dentistry becomes more expensive as we age, which stands as further confirmation that oral health generally deteriorates if you follow traditional advice. Yet entire nations around the world experience better oral health with far less problems and expense.

Let's understand *why* oral care advice is only partially accurate and generally inadequate—and how we, as individuals, can better manage our own oral health. To begin the process of sorting this out, let's talk in this chapter specifically about some of the incredible frustration caused by disagreements between dental professionals on certain topics. In particular, three topics that start with the letter "F"—and these are Flossing, Fillings, and Fluoridation.

As dentistry changed from a business of tooth extraction in the late 1800s to our modern-day idea that dentists enable us to enjoy ideal oral health, recommendations for patients' home care have not kept pace with new scientific discoveries. There is, after all, an impact—good *or* bad—that can stem from our choice of oral care products. The importance of our "daily use" strategies may make all the difference between having good oral health or continuing to experience problems. The game-changing effectiveness of home care is slowly being realized by dentists—but it has been an incredible oversight to leave this particular door into the world of mouth care products unlocked, unattended, and open to companies who may not have your oral health as a priority or concern.

Oral care companies, on the other hand, have been able to quickly understand people's collective desire for whiter teeth and they have walked decisively into this area of public need, invading it with aggressive marketing and the promotion of what can charitably be deemed a cavalcade of dubious products. Unfortunately, dentists are constant targets for "solution-based" products that do not work, created by these corporations and marketed to become the next "smoke and mirrors" phenomenon. Experienced hygienists are usually savvy to this repetitious event, but often are forced to watch as yet another unworthy product quickly becomes the newest darling of dental offices. Many oral health professionals refer to these hyped-up products and devices as dentistry's "shiny new toys," and some examples of these products from the past have included:

- **Strong fluoride gels and toothpastes.** These are many times more concentrated than the fluoride added to drinking water and were designed upon the false and never safety-tested premise that if a little fluoride is good . . . then more must be better.

- **Remineralizing toothpastes.** This product entered the dental arena in the early 2000s, prompted by companies trying to find a use for a surplus of powdered milk and some science that shows cheese can halt cavities and help mineralize teeth. These pastes were a dismal failure that caused a number of milk allergy problems—until they removed the milk and added a synergistic combination of xylitol and dilute sodium fluoride to the products.

- **Total-care pastes.** This product hit the market next with *triclosan* (now banned from toothpaste). The selling point was that this toothpaste could keep plaque away for twenty-four (24) hours. It transpired, however, that triclosan could react with the chlorine present in most water supplies to form formaldehyde on your toothbrush, and it also acts as an estrogen hormone disruptor.

- **Nano-hydroxyapatite (NHA) toothpastes.** NHA pastes were first developed for astronauts on space flights from a product that has such an affinity for fluoride that it was previously used in agriculture as a cheap and easy way to extract excess fluoride out of soil and water. Ironically, the marketing was to appeal to people looking for an alternative to fluoride toothpaste. The problem is that it did not truly repair damaged enamel but formed a layer on the outside of teeth.

- **Charcoal.** This substance has been claimed to whiten teeth by social media influencers. Its abrasive nature was not well-understood until people began to experience sensitivity and thinning enamel.

Dentists have never shown much interest in exploring the impact, benefits, or harm from the daily use of home oral care strategies. Most don't believe that cavities can reverse naturally to avoid a filling, and they insist that flossing is the key to oral health. When it comes to the use of fluoride to prevent cavities, dentistry is split between those who recommend all kinds of fluoride gels and pastes—and others who fear fluoride so much that they will never recommend a fluoride toothpaste or rinse *ever* . . . even if a patient's teeth are falling apart. You may hope that your dentist is able to recommend a personalized and ideal home care regimen for you—but usually their advice is a mixture of dental school information and industry advertising. This is why we need to explore these topics of disagreement so that you can find an ideal method of home care for your teeth—and feel empowered to enjoy the benefits of improved oral health.

TO FLOSS OR NOT TO FLOSS— THERE *IS* NO QUESTION

I have always maintained that the more you floss, the more you will *need* to floss. On the other hand, I am well aware of the floss training that hygienists receive—and the instructions that most laypersons have been given by dentists for decades. Ditching a mandatory floss regimen can be an emotional challenge, but I assure you that the best oral health I have ever seen as a dentist was at a time—and in a country—where I didn't even see or recognize any applied knowledge of floss or flossing in treatment. Instead, I saw scores of people imbued with great mouth health simply because they practiced good oral care and had sensible eating and drinking habits. This is why I have often looked for science to incontrovertibly support the act of flossing—and found instead only vague folklore and untenable dogma.

Flossing *Optional*

An effective oral care routine must do three things. It must:

- Protect you from plaque;
- Work to reverse cavities; and
- Stimulate gum health to combat gum disease.

I recommend an approach (described more comprehensively in Part Two) that involves xylitol, resilient toothbrushes, and specific oral care products, but—believe it or not—flossing is *optional*. This is because the critical flaw at the heart of flossing is that it fails to deal with the plaque-forming bacteria that float in saliva. Unless we address plaque on teeth *and* in saliva, these bacteria will drop from saliva and land on the surfaces of freshly cleaned teeth to repopulate and reinfect them. Plaque bacteria in saliva will flow into and around every surface of your mouth, entering tiny crevices in tooth enamel, going under crowns, around fillings, and deep into gum pockets—areas that are impossible to clean sufficiently with any kind of flossing string. Only through the help of products in liquid form, or xylitol—which dissolves in saliva to become a liquid—can we hope to clean around and inside these hidden areas. The idea of *not* flossing may seem shocking at first, but below is an account of the published story of Helen Rumbelow, a *Times of London* reporter who stopped flossing in 2012.

A *Times of London* Report

Helen was writing an article for *The Times of London*, and she contacted me during her search for an oral health expert who could describe the best way to floss. I explained that I have never flossed, and never recommended flossing to any patient, which was not the answer she had expected. I explained that as a dentist in Switzerland, I had seen so many healthy mouths—of patients who never flossed.

Helen had flossed for years, and despite her best efforts, had never managed to please her dental hygienist. Before she started using my strategies, she booked an appointment and asked her dentist for a numeric score to describe the status of her dental health. Her score was a six out of ten. Then Helen asked her hygienist what would happen if she gave up flossing and—as you would guess—the description was one of disaster. She listened to the gloomy description of plaque, crusty so-called *calculus* deposits under the gums, areas of bleeding, and spaces called *pockets* that would open around her teeth—virtually the complete demise of her mouth.

Learning from me, Helen began using my regimen and stopped

flossing her teeth for a month. Then she returned to her dentist for a review, without mentioning the changes she had made. To her surprise—and without prompting—her hygienist exclaimed in amazement about the significant improvements she noticed in Helen's mouth. There was no longer any bleeding and no sign of plaque or gum inflammation. Helen walked out of her appointment with a shining ten out of ten—for the first time ever.

Helen contacted the Chief of the British Oral Health Foundation and the Professor Emeritus of dental public health at University College, London. Both dentists agreed xylitol was a wonderful adjunct for oral health and that it could prevent the accumulation of plaque. They agreed people should be more aware of the power of xylitol and felt dentists simply get "bogged down" with the mechanics of dentistry. These experts also corroborated that flossing was not supported by science and was more of an ongoing legend than a science-based tool. Helen's article ignited a firestorm on both sides of the Atlantic, and the *BBC World Service* did an interview where I discussed xylitol with two eminent British dentists—who also agreed xylitol is more effective than floss.

Another article came in the summer of 2016 from Jeff Donn (a writer for the *Associated Press* wire service), where Donn asked for government records to show evidence about the need to floss for oral health. The US government acknowledged floss was never proven to be effective—something required for it to be a national guideline—and so it was removed. Donn also asked a dental school professor why there is no scientific evidence for the benefits of flossing, and the professor quipped that study results are always bad because people just "don't know how to floss *properly*." Really? So why do dentists cling to this old idea that flossing is the mainstay of oral health—when obviously it is not?

Perhaps floss sales provide financial support to the American Dental Association (ADA), but the real root of the matter is that dentists are simply wedded to their ingrained dogma on the topic. For this reason, it seems highly unlikely that your dentist will support any idea to give up flossing—but if *you* are fed up with the process or feel like a flossing failure, then maybe you can use the interval between dental visits for your *own* experiment. Most people see improvements within days and feel positive differences as they start using my strategies. You can ask your dentist why he or she has not recommended xylitol. The answer may be either that they have not yet seen "enough" studies; they perhaps have believed several inaccurate media headlines on the topic; or they have been trained by a dental school professor who thinks that you—the *patient*—should learn to floss better.

Downside of Flossing

If you are a happy flosser, be aware of concerns about *polyfluoroalkyl substances* (PFAS) lurking in most commercially sold string. These PFASs are synthetics put into consumer products since the 1950s, to help floss glide more easily between teeth. PFAS chemicals have been linked to liver damage, immune system issues, even cancer—plus the chemicals can remain in your body for *years*. We could argue the ideal time to floss is with toothpaste on your teeth—even adding additional paste to the string. Then the floss will move toothpaste between your teeth for added benefit, assuming you are using a good toothpaste. Every now and again, we all find something stuck between our teeth, and the first thing to do is to rinse with water. If this does not release and solve the problem, try a toothbrush if possible—or xylitol. My advice is to use floss only as a last resort—because, again, it appears that the *more* you floss, the more you will *need* to floss. Another concern with floss comes from the possibility that people with gum disease may unwittingly push bacteria into their blood while flossing.

This idea needs further investigation, especially since a study (published in June 2024 in the *Journal of Dental Research*) indicated that people with advanced gum disease, even young adults—who had none of the signs or factors normally associated with heart disease—had more risk for strokes and plaque buildup in their carotid arteries, three months after a deep dental cleaning.

Water Flosser or Mouthwash?

Most dentists are frustrated when patients do not floss well enough, and hygienists know that chiding us to floss is annoying. The solution for ineffective flossing arrived in dental offices as an expensive device that squirts liquid between teeth. Brilliant marketing of this equipment has convinced dentists that a *water flosser* can do a better job than string. It is interesting that dentists will regularly promote water flossing but usually ignore or even dispute the easier, safer, less expensive, and arguably more effective liquid cleaning achieved by using mouthwash.

We know plaque bacteria float in saliva, so it is easy to see that mouth cleaning will be more complete when a liquid is swished between teeth, rather than trying to remove it with a length of string—especially if your teeth are crowded or your mouth has obstacles like retainers, bridgework, crowns, or braces. The kind of liquid used as a mouthwash or in a water flosser will impact its success, so we need to understand the effect of the kind of liquid used in either case. It is fine to add salt or xylitol to a water flosser, for example, but never use bleach. Also be aware that the jet should *never* be angled into pockets, as you may risk pushing periodontal bacteria into your blood and it can prevent gum pockets from healing. If you have periodontal pockets, stop using the device until your pockets heal (using the strategies described in Part Two—no water or string flossing required). I will discuss the misunderstanding about mouthwash's effect on oral bacteria in Part Two, along with other details about the products that comprise my Complete Mouth Care System™.

So, Are Fillings Full of It?

A small filling sounds like an easy fix, but before you agree to treatment, consider there are ways to prompt cavities to heal naturally. Most dentists agree that a small cavity in enamel can be reversed with correct care, and doing this offers the opportunity to preserve a valuable pristine tooth. Even a cavity into dentin may reverse, so ideally, ask your dentist if you can delay any cavity treatment for three (3) to six (6) months. This should give you time to improve the way you are looking after your teeth in this time interval. Even if the original cavity does not completely heal, and your tooth still requires a filling, any drilling will be safer for the tooth and less likely to damage the nerve inside the tooth, after three or more months on my strategies. A dentist who values teeth should be thrilled if a cavity has reversed itself, and you should be happy to have maintained a pristine, uncut tooth.

Some dentists, however, have a more flippant attitude to fillings, and are often fixated on the notion that all cavities need immediate repair with a filling—and they don't feel any concern about negative consequences. Most cavity diagnoses are subjective to some degree—and always remember that once a tooth has been drilled, filled, or sealed, these treatments cannot be reversed, and natural healing will no longer be possible. Dental marketing can be aggressive, sensitive diagnostic detection equipment can create false positive results, and research shows many cavities are filled that could have healed with correct care. In some offices, the dental staff are choreographed to work as a team and to consider how much insurance money is available for your dental care. *More* treatment is not better for your mouth, so be a wary shopper.

White fillings are made of plastic, and they attract sticky cavity-forming bacteria to their edges, which is why they are often called *plaque magnets*. This is a problem in a mouth where saliva is acidic or when a patient is not using effective home care strategies. In such cases, white fillings will appear to need repair and refilling every ten (10) to fifteen (15) years. This means that if you decide to change an old silver-amalgam filling for a new white one, you will likely need frequent replacements, and each one can endanger the life of your tooth.

When a tooth's nerve dies, it will need a root canal and crown, or an extraction and implant. Many patients do not consider all these facts before agreeing to the replacement of their old silver fillings, and end up enduring repeated fillings, dead teeth, root canals, and

Stop vs. Prevent

A *filling* is dental material that blocks holes in teeth, like a patch in the pavement—and this can make the surface smooth again, help your tooth to look good, and improve its function for eating and chewing. A filling stops damage from progressing through your tooth, but unless the bacteria that cause these cavities are addressed, *more* cavities will form in your mouth in other teeth or around the edges of this original filling.

On the other hand, if you decide to take immediate action and eradicate the cavity-forming bacteria with the strategies described up ahead in Part Two, you will improve the condition of your mouth to prevent *future* cavities—and potentially reverse the original cavity at the same time.

There is a difference between treatments that stop—and strategies that *prevent*—cavities and gum disease. Most people understand that fillings stop cavities, and that dental cleanings can slow gum disease, but neither treatment can prevent a future cavity or gum problems. To highlight this important distinction, let's consider a scenario where your dentist finds an early cavity in your tooth. He or she may suggest that it be filled immediately, but sometimes you may be given the chance to do something that can seem a little unusual at first glance. Some dentists, especially if you have a perfect and as-yet unfilled tooth, may suggest they wait and see if this cavity deteriorates between then and your next visit.

Why would you ever wait for a cavity to grow? Instead, you can use the specific oral care products and strategies that will be explained in detail in Part Two to dazzle your dentist by healing this tooth and preventing its progression—*before* your next appointment. It makes no sense to continue using the strategies that allowed this cavity to happen in the first place. Anyone with a cavity must change *something* in the way they care for their teeth and alter the direction of the disease. This new strategy would be called *preventive*, as it addresses the future as well as helping to heal the initial cavity.

Similarly, if you follow dentistry's traditional advice to brush and floss and have regular cleanings, then you can wait and see if you end up with gum disease—the dental woes experienced by ninety-six percent (96%) of older Americans. Or you can decide to take control of your oral health and avoid the situation that I will describe in the following story.

An employee of the American Dental Association (ADA) contacted me to explain that for forty years, he had habitually brushed, flossed, and routinely gone for professional cleanings every six months. Despite his meticulous approach to oral care, he had developed periodontal gum disease—and now blamed his family genes. The fact is that cavities and periodontal gum disease are bacterial diseases—transferred in droplets of saliva as we talk, kiss, and hug within our circles of family and friends.

For this gentleman, disease bacteria likely transferred from family members, and the disease may have been accelerated by inherited habits, or an inherited anatomy such as a jaw or lip shape, that could make it hard for him to close his mouth, making him a mouth breather, drying his saliva, and putting him at more risk for gum disease. You can also have a genetic disposition that puts you at *more* risk for gum disease, but the problem is always initially caused by plaque bacteria. An effective strategy will combat these bacteria and control them, since we know periodontal disease is preventable.

This individual had experienced sufficient protection from his careful brushing and flossing to suffice for most of his life, but as he aged, this traditional form of oral care was insufficient to protect him or prevent the bacteria that ignited the condition of gum disease in his midlife years. So, knowing this, why would you wait for periodontal gum disease to happen to you?

crowns. This is why many people I know wish they could reconsider their decision to replace amalgam fillings, in light of how their respective stories ended.

Silver amalgams are more durable than white ones, but there is concern about the mercury they contain. There is some disagreement about the absolute toxicity of silver mercury fillings, but most dentists agree that they pose the highest risk as the amalgam is being used to fill a cavity and when it is being drilled out in the process of removal. Some studies have shown it can take seventeen (17) years for our body to naturally detoxify mercury amalgam particles that may have been swallowed or left in your mouth during the placement of a silver filling.

If you have fillings from decades ago, your body may have already detoxified itself and you need to ask if the dangers from replacement are a desirable option. Studies with autopsy indicate that a healthy person can naturally detoxify a total of ten (10) to twelve (12) silver fillings over a lifetime. Everyone with silver fillings should know the damages of artificial whitening products and peroxides, which cause mercury to be released as a gas from any silver fillings you may have in your mouth.

Sealants are a plastic coating made with a material that resembles the white plastic used in fillings, but with a thinner consistency, so it flows into cracks and gaps in teeth. Sealants are frequently suggested to parents as a treatment to block the crevices in young children's teeth, a treatment that dentistry considers useful to try and prevent cavities for a few years. In molar teeth, sealants play a defensive role and block up the grooves where cavities could form in a decay-prone mouth. But cavity-forming bacteria are only blocked from entering the grooves of teeth with this superficial plastic glue. Usually, five (5) to ten (10) years later, the cavity-forming bacteria that have remained active in the saliva of a cavity-prone child will cause new damage around the edges of these sealants, resulting in a bigger area of decay and the need for even larger fillings.

Recurrent decay is the name given to this continuing cavity infection in a mouth. Xylitol has the power to stop recurrent decay for children and adults within a year, by eliminating cavity-forming bacteria in saliva and promoting healthy bacteria. When a mouth is free of cavity-forming bacteria, cavities cannot occur—with or without a sealant. In the 1980s, xylitol studies showed how the regular use of xylitol could protect children from cavities as effectively as sealants—over a ten-year period in children ages six (6) to sixteen (16). Longer-term studies, however—if they had been done, or if there was any interest in a retrospective study—would certainly show xylitol outperforming sealants, because in a decay-prone mouth sealants fail during the teenage years, but xylitol promotes healthy bacteria and eliminates plaque proactively for several years, even if the regular use of xylitol ends.

If a child has a healthy mouth and no sign of decay, then a sealant may be an even *worse* idea because they stop good bacteria from gaining access to molar crevices, which is a natural habitat and secure foothold for them. Sealants were developed before we had any understanding of good mouth bacteria, and today we know that forty percent (40%) of bacteria in an adult mouth becomes established in childhood—and that the crevices in a child's molar teeth operate as vehicles to carry good bacteria into an adult mouth.

Remarkably, it appears that the impact of sealants on a child's digestive health has never been studied, especially with respect to the possible development of gluten intolerances. The mission of the American Academy of Pediatric Dentistry (AAPD) is to seal every child's tooth in America, despite the risks from exposure to micro-plastic molecules and chemicals in the plastic, along with changes that sealants potentially cause to a child's developing mouth and digestive bacteria.

Beyond Fillings—A Dental Implant

You could be forgiven for thinking implants are like a birthday gift—an easy way to have a new tooth, or set of teeth, to replace the ones that caused you trouble, after the point in time when a filling is no longer possible. It is shocking to discover that, in America, twenty-five percent (25%) of seniors by age seventy-four have lost all their natural teeth and require tooth replacements.

When you explore implants, they are often described in flowery language that makes patients imagine something very different from a screw drilled into the jawbone with a fake tooth glued on top. You may think implants are a solution to your dental problems, and that after a little sedation, you will simply wake up to a gorgeous new set of teeth. Certainly, they can dramatically change your mouth but realize that any infection that damaged your natural teeth will be even more likely to ruin your implant, unless you make changes to ensure that your mouth is as healthy as possible before the change.

Sometimes an implant will replace a missing tooth—one that never grew or was lost in an accident. Implants may also be suggested following tooth loss from gum disease or when fillings wrecked your tooth's structure. Consider that gum disease can happen to implants—and if you have plaque, it can cause worse damage to an implant. In a healthy mouth, a natural tooth attaches to the jawbone and derives strength and support from a special periodontal fiber attachment.

The problem is that implants do not integrate in the same way with your jawbone. The periodontal barrier fibers create a defensive barrier around a natural tooth but not around an implant. Select a dentist with experience if you are having an implant, as minimal mistakes can lead to failure and fracture of this new tooth, or the loss of the supporting screw. Implants cause more trouble for people who smoke or vape, and for the elderly, and those who take medications—particularly the kind of pharmaceuticals used to help treat anxiety, depression, rheumatoid arthritis, and/or acid reflux.

Most implants will last for ten (10) or more years, but their maintenance is challenging, particularly if you are someone who relies on regular cleanings. Particles of titanium can easily be scratched off the implant and your hygienist should use a special (albeit *expensive*) cleaning tool with a softer blade designed for implants. Titanium particles are sometimes associated with chronic inflammation in the jaw and symptoms of autoimmune disease in susceptible individuals. Internet fears have persuaded many people to avoid a root canal in favor of an extraction and implant. My advice is to consider every way to preserve a natural tooth, even if this involves a root canal and crown, before deciding on an implant. Extraction will cause a loss of connection between the tooth's supporting periodontal fibers and the brain—something that may reduce release in the brain of an enzyme called *orexin*, a neuropeptide that affects both vision and cognitive health and has an impact on the body's sleep-wake cycle.

Minimally Invasive Dentistry

Good dentists should always be concerned about the potential damage that can be caused to a tooth's nerves whenever a cavity is drilled or filled. Nerves can die during the removal and replacement of a filling, or if a crown is made to cover a tooth, but often it takes time for these problems to become obvious. Sometimes it can take ten or more years before you are aware that the nerve has died in your tooth, alerted by a sudden throbbing pain that signals dead tooth problems. This risk is not generally understood by patients, but in the 1970s, a number of forward-thinking dentists started to consider how fillings and other treatments could be performed to avoid these drilling risks, and they looked for ways to fill teeth with care and avoid damage to either the tooth nerve or its essential structure—a practice known as *minimally invasive dentistry*.

The group eventually split into two:

1. Some dentists formed the Academy of Biomimetic Dentistry (AOBMD), a group of dentists who share skills and experiences with each other, working to create the most *ideal* fillings—ones that stop cavities with the least amount of drilling and tooth trauma. AOBMD dentists work to preserve the life of teeth with minimally invasive techniques. These dentists attend endless classes after graduation and learn exacting filling techniques that mimic nature, working with fiberglass and ceramic—extremely strong materials with less potential to harm the inside of the tooth. They use computers to design fillings with the least amount of drilling and tooth damage. Originally, this process was called Chairside Economical Restoration of Aesthetic Ceramics (CERAC)—but today the techniques are even more effective, and they continue to raise the public's expectations of good restorative dental care.

2. Another group focused instead on teaching patients how best to prevent cavities in the first place, by changing their risk for decay. They assessed the patients' daily habits, diet, and home care

with a program called Caries Management By Risk Assessment (CAMBRA). In recent years it appears some of these ideals have changed—as leaders have developed more associations with oral care companies. I am shocked to see CAMBRA proponents recommend bleach and concentrated levels of stannous fluoride—strategies that I do not endorse because of the potential harm they can do to teeth and mouth bacteria.

The world needs a dental organization that embodies minimally invasive dentistry and ideal motives. This organization should teach effective do-it-yourself (DIY) home care for individuals and promote non-drill techniques to heal tooth decay that can be used by dental and medical professionals for children and adults. The mission of this organization should be to eradicate the pain, fear, and ongoing disease that is still prevalent globally. The focus should be on the development of an approach that is useful for rural and underserved areas around the world. I am proud to have helped support one such fledgling organization at its inception, but I believe we need more robust change across America and a wider acceptance of the practical answers outlined in this book that provide smart and painless dental help for children and adults.

FLUORIDATION—CONTROVERSIAL, AND CONFUSING

Is fluoride toxic to our brain—and if so, why do dentists want everyone to drink it, have teeth coated with it, and brush with toothpaste containing it? The actual word *fluoride* has created so much fear and confusion that some people choose to let their teeth decay, crack, and even die—rather than rinse and spit with a fluoride mouthwash. This repulsion is so generalized in the world of alternative health that oral care corporations like the Colgate-Palmolive Company—reviled *because* they make fluoride toothpastes—have purchased trusted "non-fluoride" brands (like Tom's of Maine) so they can blithely continue to sell products and reach a base of customers who would never knowingly purchase a Colgate-affiliated product.

This fluoride debate was unwittingly seeded in 1901 by a newly graduated dentist named Frederick McKay. He had noticed some of the patients in his Colorado Springs, Colorado-based practice had teeth that were malformed and discolored. With help from famous dental expert Dr. G. V. Black (who we already discussed in Chapter One), the two men studied these teeth under a microscope and saw that the discoloration was caused by gaps in the enamel where it had not formed properly. They shared this discovery at dental meetings around the world and many others had seen similarly malformed teeth. In every case, the teeth in question were amazingly strong and without cavities.

Fluorosis—What It Is, and How It Happens

Today we understand more about these tooth malformations, which occur if children under the age of six (6) drink fluoridated water at the time their adult teeth are forming. Cells in the child's jaw—called *ameloblasts*—make tooth enamel, but they are extremely sensitive to fluoride. If these cells die, the adult tooth forms but gaps can occur in the enamel where the ameloblasts died. The defects usually show themselves as white lines or spots on tooth surfaces, but in severe cases they occur as brown patches. This problem is called *fluorosis*, and it can *only* happen to children under the age of six, *while* their adult teeth are forming.

Dr. McKay studied the problem for twenty years and was finally convinced these malformations were the result of something occurring naturally in his local water supply. This is why Dr. McKay arranged for the water of Colorado Springs to be re-routed—and within ten years, children in his area were no longer developing malformed teeth. This could have been the end of the story, except that there were four hundred (400) other cities in America that had reported similar issues to the United States Public Health Service. H. Trendly Dean was the government official tasked with investigating the severity of these tooth defects, and in 1931 he began to grade them as mild, moderate, and severe. By 1934, he had made an association between the severity of the damage and the amount of fluoride these children were drinking in their naturally fluoridated water supply. Dean showed that the more fluoride they drank, the more severe the pitting and enamel discoloration in the tooth surfaces—a condition that he called enamel *fluorosis*.

The immediate goal was to find a way to remove fluoride from drinking water supplies where it was naturally too abundant. Developments over the next fifteen (15) years, however, redirected this plan, and a new idea developed—to put fluoride *into* drinking water supplies of cities where fluoride was absent. Dean's mindset started to change as he began to compare the number of cavities in children's teeth with the amount of fluorosis in them, as he looked at children's teeth in the twenty-one (21) American states where problems had been reported.

Fluoridation of Water

Fluoride is one of the most common elements in nature, and it is found in varying concentrations and in many soils and ground water in the United States and other countries around the world. Again, H. Trendly Dean had discovered that when there was a concentration of one (1) to two (2) parts per million of fluoride naturally occurring in the drinking water supplies, fluorosis of teeth was generally mild, and the number of cavities was low. Dean proposed adjusting water to what he called "an ideal concentration" of fluoride so that drinking this water would help teeth to resist cavities.

Cavities at this time were viewed as an epidemic problem in the United States, and particularly for military recruits who were being enlisted amid the rising tensions that preempted World War Two. By 1940, a rapid twist had occurred in the fluoride investigation; from the consideration of water supplies with too much fluoride, public discussion and goals of the issue moved over to the seemingly contradictory notion that water could instead be called *deficient* in fluoride. It is interesting that this was also the moment when an unusual fluorosis problem surfaced in the state of Arkansas.

The *Twist* in the Story

Fluorosis had been observed within communities in the city of Baux-ite, Arkansas, located close to the Aluminum Company Of America (ALCOA), where testing showed that the levels were fifteen (15) times higher than Dean had pronounced safe for teeth. For years, the fluoride that was produced as a waste product by aluminum manufacture had been sold by ALCOA as a registered pesticide across the USA—until the advent of stronger chemical pesticides. ALCOA became involved in the government investigations because of the high fluoride levels around its manufacturing plant, but soon thereafter Dean became interested in the idea that fluoride should be adjusted and even added to cure a "deficiency" in all of America's water supplies, and ALCOA soon began to sell their industry excess fluoride to water authorities.

Records show ALCOA's engineers and attorneys, and one of their stockholders and founders—the famed American industri-alist Andrew Mellon—began to develop connections and sponsor research at the Carnegie-Mellon Institute (the institution which in 1967 merged with the Carnegie Institute of Technology to become today's Carnegie-Mellon University in Pittsburgh). The Carne-gie-Mellon Institute was ideally positioned for these fluoride studies as a part of its mission to support comprehensive scientific studies that would serve industry and benefit mankind through the devel-opment of industry.

By 1945, fluoride supplementation of water began in the popu-lous city of Grand Rapids, Michigan; and by 1951, water fluoridation had become an official public health policy in the United States. In 1952, concerned scientists argued at the Delaney Committee Con-gressional Hearings that fluoride levels in drinking water in the United States were too high, especially for children and people with diabetes or kidney disease. This was also when the fire of distrust concerning fluoridation was sparked, and it has blazed in the dental profession ever since. The end of the story was that Dean became the first director of the National Institute of Dental Research. Finger pointing continues, even at a political level, questioning all the legal and institutional fluoride decisions—back to the government investigation in the 1930s. The American Dental Association has consistently backed water fluoridation, and dentists are generally trained to believe in the wonders of fluoride.

A Lack of Trust

Personally, I join the dentists who vehemently oppose water fluoridation and question why our water supplies are still fluoridated in the twenty-first century. Indeed, a report issued by the US government in the summer of 2024 indicates that fluoride at twice the recommended limit in drinking water has now been linked to lower IQ levels in children worldwide. There are non-fluoridated cities and countries where they enjoy the same levels of oral health as those that are fluoridated. There has never been any regard to fluoride's interaction with materials in local plumbing, or pharmaceuticals and chemicals found in modern water supplies. At a City Hall meeting in Austin to vote on local water fluoridation, it stunned me to watch as valid concerns were rebutted by bogus, non-scientific arguments from ADA spokespeople. Do the supporters of water fluoridation have any demonstrable knowledge of fluoride's dubious history or the effectiveness of topical products? I think newly graduated dentists may not, but perhaps this may be the generation to challenge the ADA and question *why* they are still so heavily invested in fluoride.

Fluoride offers no benefit to baby teeth, and young children are the ones at risk for fluorosis if they drink fluoridated water before the age of six. In the 1970s, in areas without fluoride, parents were encouraged to supplement with fluoride drops. I gave my oldest children this fluoride "supplementation" in the suggested dose, but when their adult teeth grew into their respective mouths by around the time that they each were seven years old, they had brown marks and rough surfaces on them as is commonly seen in cases of moderate fluorosis. As a dentist, I myself was ignorant of this potential for fluorosis damage as recently as 1980. This is why we should allow people to choose a method of adding fluoride if they desire. In Switzerland, fluoride is offered in salt, and consumers can select fluoridated or non-fluoridated salt—just as in the United States some salt is iodized. In addition, we see that milk fluoridation occurs presently in parts of Eastern Europe, China, and South America.

Since fluoride is naturally occurring in many water supplies, it ends up in many foods we consume—and especially in many drinks. Excessive amounts of fluoride should always be avoided, especially by children under the age of six who are at risk for fluorosis. Most brewed teas—*iced* tea, in particular—have high concentrations of fluoride. Raisins, grapes, and wine also have a high fluoride content. Potatoes and other foods have fluoride in them. We used to think that fluoride was rendered inactive by milk, but this is not correct. It is simply that when fluoride and milk—or *any* calcium-rich food, for that matter—are consumed together, less fluoride will be absorbed into the bloodstream from ninety percent (90%) percent to about sixty percent (60%).

Topical Use Only

If the fluoride antics of industry and government make you angry, you may be surprised that I now want to discuss the *benefits* of fluoride. Many who fiercely oppose fluoride will never use a topical drop—either in a rinse or a toothpaste. The key to effective dental home care is to recognize the important difference between treatments to stop a cavity and strategies that prevent one from forming. To illustrate this in the context of fluoride, we can consider how acidity softens a tooth by pulling minerals from its surface. Then cavity-forming bacteria enter the porosities in the tooth and begin to undermine its structure. At some point, the tooth caves in and creates a cavity. We have discussed how a filling can stop a cavity from progressing by repairing the hole in the tooth—but to *prevent* a cavity, three things must occur:

1. Mouth acidity must be controlled;

2. Cavity-forming bacteria must be eradicated; and

3. Lost minerals from a tooth's surface must be replenished.

The only part of this preventive sequence where fluoride can contribute is to help speed up the deposition of lost minerals on the tooth's surface. If minerals deposit often and fast enough, this may completely combat demineralization. On the other hand, fluoride does not change the mouth's acidity, and the compound of fluoride that I recommend—*sodium fluoride*—has no effect on bacteria. This is why the use of fluoride for prevention should always be paired with xylitol strategies to control mouth acidity and support a healthy mix of mouth bacteria.

Remineralizing with Fluoride

The benefits from brushing and rinsing—with a low concentration of sodium fluoride toothpaste or a 0.05% level of sodium fluoride mouth rinse—can help reverse tooth damage for adults and children over the age of six (who can rinse and spit effectively, that is). Regular use of this specific type of fluoride, at this specific dilute concentration, can improve weak, sensitive, or damaged teeth. Personal friends of mine are doctors who specialize in thyroid, Alzheimer's, and enzyme conditions, and who have tested to ensure that this kind of topical fluoride use is not absorbed through the mouth. They concluded, after twenty years of observation, that the risks were negligible or none, and the benefits from topical fluoride drastically improved their patients' oral health—and even their systemic health.

Why refuse the benefits of remineralization in exchange for the possible toxicity of white or silver fillings, the pain and suffering or root canals, lost teeth, and health consequences from damaged teeth and need for implants? This is like a drowning person who refuses a life preserver because they dislike the texture of the fabric from which it has been made. This is why I have not included the word "future"—as a final or fourth "F" of dentistry. Change is coming that may allow development of personalized equipment, so patients can measure and monitor their own mouth health.

CONCLUSION

In this chapter, we looked at three areas of dental care where controversy abounds. We investigated the nooks and crannies of *flossing*, a care practice which I think is largely unnecessary if you approach oral health with more complete and effective methods. We explored the topic of *fillings*, and their need, which I believe can be dramatically reduced by effective self-directed oral care applied at home. And we considered the topic of *fluoridation*, and why some fluoride can be useful—but how there are extreme differences between the various kinds of fluoride; how concentration levels matter; and how consuming it presents us with dangers, though we can safely enjoy its benefits with the topical application of a toothpaste or through use of a dilute sodium fluoride rinse.

The overall secret should now be obvious—we *all* need to take charge of our own oral health. We need to divorce ourselves from dependence on a system that appears so influenced by other unspoken goals—and unseen agendas. Simple strategies can help you to care for your teeth, including the use of xylitol that has provided decades of positive experiences in other countries—and which remains at the core of my system.

My general advice, therefore, is to find a dentist you trust—possibly even through "virtual" tele-dentistry sessions that can be achieved at home—and ensure, through that dialogue, that you have regular *evaluations* to ensure you are moving in the direction of gum, tooth, and mouth health. Saliva testing, periodic X-rays, and cancer screening are always helpful, but try to sidestep or ask if you can delay traditional preventive treatments. You will have to consider your feelings toward flossing, sealants, small fillings, frequent cleanings, and strong fluoride treatments—which, if you take my advice and embrace my system, you will no longer need.

5

*D*ental Science + Common Sense = Something to Chew On

The problem with common sense is that it's not so common.

—François-Marie Arouet (pen name: Voltaire)

According to a recent World Health Organization (WHO) report, untreated cavities and gum disease affect over 3.5 billion adults and 514 million children across the globe. Most readers, especially in the United States, assume that their fellow Americans generally have good teeth. However, clinical observation and insurance industry statistics show that the volume of treatment and disease rates in this country are extraordinarily high—with a staggering ninety-six percent (96%) of seniors forced to endure a spiral of dental expenses for fillings that need repair; teeth that die and need extraction; cleanings that become more invasive and complicated at each dental visit; and gum health that deteriorates to the point when it may require the surgical removal of skin from the roof of the mouth to graft or sew into areas where it has disappeared.

All these horrors are simply the consequence of an ongoing but preventable disease in our mouth that has been allowed to fester and attack our teeth and gums. The treatments that your dentist can provide will stop any pain and may delay the loss of your natural teeth, but it would all cease to be necessary if the bacterial disease and imbalances in your mouth were adequately controlled by your daily home care and routines.

CAN A DENTIST STOP CAVITIES . . . AND OTHER DENTAL PROBLEMS?

Many patients assume their dentist knows how to stop cavities. If, however, you have had the unpleasant and costly experience of ongoing dental treatments—fillings, repairs, crowns, and years of cleanings, possibly with the unfortunate ending of extracted teeth and implants—you may question how this happened. Perhaps you have been indoctrinated to believe it was your fault, due either to a failure to follow some fancy flossing instructions or because you missed a dental cleaning appointment.

You will begin to unravel the truth, however, if you ask yourself the following question instead: *Can a dentist stop cavities and other dental problems—or is it up to an individual?*

The answer will surface if you dive into the science of cavities and gum disease and notice how these infections are improved or worsened by the variable daily conditions in our mouths. A dentist can fix dental damage *after* it has happened, but she or he cannot control the daily conditions in your mouth—and it is these that increase or decrease our risk for cavities and gum disease. Consider a similar situation—can your doctor prevent you from catching a cold? Obviously not, but your doctor can advise you how to manage your body's defense systems so you can have a better chance at avoiding any sickness. In the same way, the only person with the power to stop cavities and gum disease is *you*—and just like preventing a cold, the best strategies are defensive ones.

The second question we should ask is: *Why is there so much dental disease?* Some professionals say it's because patients don't floss enough, while others blame too much sugar in our diet. Plaque and sugar are certainly a part of this problem, but cavities and gum disease are infections sparked by specific bacteria that can fester on dirty toothbrushes and become worse if habits and bad care choices dry out our mouths or allow teeth to become porous. Dentists are trained to fix dental problems after they occur, but if you want to stop dental problems and enjoy a cavity-free future, then it is *you* who must become empowered and be ready to take charge of your own mouth health by modifying your daily habits and care, to protect your teeth from harm. Sometimes it is difficult to grasp the reality that dental treatments *cannot* prevent cavities or gum disease, even if you have your teeth professionally cleaned several times a year. The answer lies in how you care for your teeth every day—before, after, and between dental appointments.

This brings us to the final question: *Why is there so much disagreement about the most effective home care strategies for oral health?* With social media pressures and industry marketing, there are more questions than answers when it comes to selecting the best or most helpful products for daily care. Because of this, we have some dentists who proclaim that it is impossible to expect complete protection from cavities and gum disease, and so they have no faith that teeth and gums can heal naturally. This pessimism often develops during dental school education, and it can be perpetuated by dental office culture.

Remember, of course, to never blame yourself or your age for dental problems. Instead, let's look at the status of oral health in some other countries where oral health outcomes are superior to America, and consider some of their approaches—at a national level, within families, and as individuals.

From Nation to Nation

In countries that enjoy the healthiest teeth, dental education has been able to teach the concept of how children's dental problems begin as cavity-forming bacteria transfer from the mouths of parents to their children and then from child to child. Cavity-forming bacteria can travel in droplets of saliva as people talk, hug, or kiss their babies and family members, or share eating utensils and living spaces together. Xylitol can eliminate this bacterial transmission by cleaning the saliva.

This is why parents are encouraged to enjoy a regular xylitol regimen during pregnancy and after the baby is born. In some countries, xylitol gum is distributed in preschool for the same reason—to reduce the transfer of cavity-forming bacteria from child to child at this important stage of tooth development. Studies show that children who grow up in this preventive culture will have eighty-five percent (85%) to ninety-two percent (92%) less incidence of cavities.

At an international level, oral health is computed by counting how many decayed, missing, or filled teeth are found in examined mouths. Using this measurement, America is in tenth place globally, with Denmark as number one, and then Germany, Finland, and Sweden as the top four countries on this list. As mentioned, xylitol is endorsed by the dental associations of all these top countries, and the Danish population have almost perfect teeth—with less than a quarter of a tooth showing any decay, either in baby or adult teeth. Remember also the important fact that the health of baby teeth will go on to impact the health of developing adult teeth.

Family

Today, we understand how bacteria transfer from person to person—from a parent's mouth to a child, and even jumping from the surfaces of a five-year-old's baby teeth to that of their new adult teeth as they enter and grow in the child's mouth. Family oral health is important, and parents—through sheer proximity—will automatically pass healthy or harmful bacteria to the mouths and teeth of their children.

Many people are surprised that adult teeth enter toward the back of a child's mouth as early as his or her fifth birthday. Many of these new adult teeth develop cavities—often within twelve months, and even before a child's sixth birthday—simply because the parents were unaware how to effectively manage cavity-forming bacteria with daily home care. This is why it is also good to use effective strategies for family members: before the birth of a baby, as babies' first teeth are breaking through their gums during childhood, and as children grow into adolescence—and while they are developing a full complement of new adult teeth. These changes will make a dramatic difference to the dental health of families, but particularly for those who already have a painful history of bad teeth.

Individuals

Cavities and chronic periodontal gum disease are common but completely *preventable* dental problems. With effective daily care, you can enjoy the benefits of oral health and lessen your need for dental treatments and interventions. Of course, the earlier we start, the better our chance of success. Current statistics show that two percent (2%) of the United States adult population have no teeth, while ninety-six percent (96%) have fillings, cavities, and chronic gum disease by their retirement age. The size of a filling usually increases each time it is replaced, which means that over the years fillings will cover more tooth surfaces. Eventually, most fillings will be replaced with full-coverage crowns—and, unfortunately, all this ongoing dental work can cause nerve damage, killing the tooth and leading to the next potential problem—a root canal or extraction.

The number of initially preventable and reversable fillings that are considered *normal* for American adults is between ten (10) and twelve (12) per person. This illustrates how inadequate the widely accepted "brush and floss" advice has been over the long term—and why you should seriously consider other methods, even if you see them as supplemental. The key is to avoid the downhill spiral that usually begins with a small filling or simple treatment. Why? The reason is because that dental work will likely deteriorate a decade later and then become a progressive need for repairs amid worsening oral health—a situation so common that many dentists believe it is merely an unavoidable consequence of age. By using my strategies, however, you will be able to prove that belief *wrong*.

Here are three actions you can take immediately:

1. **Control the amount of daily damage that your teeth experience from tooth-destructive habits.** What are these habits? It begins

with eating and drinking. Teeth are damaged every day by a variety of our all-too-human "tooth destructive" routines and habits. Unless we discover a way to compensate for this damage, our teeth will gradually become weaker and at more risk for decay, and our gums will slowly deteriorate and become vulnerable to disease. Similar damage can result from habits that involve constant sipping (even *water*); the smoking of cigars and/or cigarettes; vaping; chewing tobacco; continuous snacking (especially candy, sugary cookies, crackers, carbohydrates, and processed foods); or from going to sleep at night without appropriately cleaning your teeth.

2. **Provide your mouth with resting intervals *between* meals, when you do not eat or drink anything.** Why do this? You do it so that the saliva in your mouth is given the chance to interact with your teeth and gums. Saliva carries all the minerals necessary to rebuild—and *repair*—tooth enamel and immune cells that help heal your gums. These periods of healing are our mouth's daily *repair* experiences, and they must be long enough and frequent enough to balance out the damage created by the *negative* experiences that come from our daily tooth-destructive habits.

Foods that damage our teeth are the aforementioned sugary, acidic, and carbohydrate-containing foods. Some cause a direct acidic attack, while others cause acidic damage indirectly as sugars turn to acids. Surprisingly, the severity of this damage is not influenced by the *amount* of sugar you eat, and two grains will potentially cause as much mouth damage as a pound of sugary pudding. The amount of tooth damage caused will depend specifically on the length of time acids attack your teeth. This means that damage will be influenced by the stickiness of food, as this prolongs the time sugar sits in your mouth. Moreover, acidic mouth damage extends for an hour after your last bite of food, but once this acidity has been neutralized, then your saliva will begin to deposit minerals and repair any damage caused by foods.

Most dentists suggest it takes an hour for our saliva to clear acidity after eating, but with a xylitol regimen we can shorten this to a matter of minutes and turn this hour of damage into an hour of healing. If you eat meals four (4) times a day, you can turn the post-meal hours into four (4) hours of healing. This, combined with nighttime healing, may be a sufficient change to maintain mouth health. The more time you allow for healing, of course, the more help you will have for your gums and teeth.

This also explains why snacking and sipping habits are so dangerous, as they continue to compound the amount of time your teeth are being damaged. Their presence in your daily life delays the end of your eating and/or drinking times. You get caught in a vicious cycle—as you graze on just one more piece of food or take another sip of drink, your actions serve to restart the mouth's "one hour after eating" period of damage. Consider the number of eating or drinking sessions you have each day, and the length of after-meal coffees, snacks, or extended sipping. Add these numbers and see how much time you spend each day damaging your mouth health. For someone who eats four (4) meals and one (1) snack, your teeth could be under attack for at least five (5) hours a day!

The ideal is to keep meals and snacks to confined sessions and then cease eating and drinking for an hour or longer. In addition, ending snacks and meals with xylitol (see Part Two for more detail on this topic) will stimulate a flow of extra-healing saliva. This can be particularly beneficial if you allow this saliva to coat your mouth for an hour or two in this interval between eating and drinking.

Xylitol is an ally that helps us shorten periods of tooth damage and turn our mouth environment from damaging acidity into one of healing. Instead of waiting an hour for acidity to normalize after meals, a xylitol mint or piece of gum instantly stops the damage and starts the healing of your gums and teeth. When you end every meal or snack with xylitol, assuming you eat four meals and one snack per day, you can create five hours of healing rather than damage—and this can create a dramatic shift in mouth health.

3. **Support the goal of creating a positive balance between the amount of healing our mouth experiences versus the amount of damage it experiences daily.** How? Well, we have the power to shorten any periods of daily damage by rinsing our mouth with water or some tooth-protective drink, ending meals with tooth-protective foods, or using xylitol. Then if you choose to not sip or snack, and if we consume foods that support salivary health (nutrition for saliva health will be discussed in Part Two), we can extend the length of these daily periods of healing and help our teeth and gums become healthier. Good daily tooth care, with the right choice of oral care products, should help support and *speed up* this healing process—while, at the same time, it *slows down* mineral loss during times of damage.

CONCLUSION

Certainly, dentists are not purposefully withholding information, and most patients agree that dentists are some of the most conscientious and caring physicians who want only the best for their patients. That said, be aware that it is difficult for a dentist to recommend an ideal method of care for you—because most dentists have no long-term experience with one product or system. Many learn about home care in dental school, taught by salespeople from product companies, and today many dental offices are integrated groups working under the umbrella of a bigger business. This is why it is vital for you to be empowered and *know* about your dental problems and available solutions—including the option of reversing a cavity or gum disease at home, by yourself, with the strategies and products that will be discussed in Part Two of this book.

By now, I hope you are excited by this idea and that you feel ready to take new steps toward oral health. And so, let's move on to Part Two—and into a world of empowerment for you and a future of happier and healthier teeth and gums.

PART TWO

The Complete Mouth Care System™

6

$\mathscr{T}$he Tooth and Nothing but the Tooth— My System, Step by Step

To put everything in balance is good,
to put everything in harmony is better.

—Victor Hugo

This chapter will give you step-by-step instructions for my Complete Mouth Care System™. It is a method that can help anyone with adult teeth achieve an improvement in their oral health—often at surprising speed. It is a protocol that requires the frequent use of: small amounts of an oral health sugar called *xylitol* (which will be described in more detail in Chapter 7); three different mouth rinses; and—while using a special kind of toothbrush—an applied regimen of brushing your teeth and gums *consistently* with a specific kind of toothpaste.

As with a musical score that has been written to create a delicate harmony or an architecture blueprint that has been designed to ensure a sturdily erected office building, this system of home dental care works best if you have a firm command of the core concepts—and understand that success depends on using an exact technique along with specific products. I call this my "Three-S" approach, and that is what we will explore together next.

THE "THREE-S" APPROACH
TO BETTER MOUTH HEALTH

Most of us already know that in every grocery and drug store there are seemingly endless choices for oral care products that claim to solve dental problems. Sensitivity gels, whitening pastes, and rinses for bad breath or gum disease are among those products that have all been specifically designed to "treat" your symptoms, but that do nothing for the deeper concern—the fact that your mouth is out of balance. By way of comparison, the products that I recommend work together in a harmonious way to promote overall mouth health. Today we have bacterial testing that can show how my system—developed and refined over years of practical application with my patients—supports *good* mouth bacteria, while reducing *harmful* ones. Through a strategic blend of what I call my "Three-S" approach—Synergy, Sequencing, Success—I am confident that you will be equipped with the winning formula when it comes to daily use of these far more effective products in the promotion of a sustainably healthy and comfortable mouth.

Synergy

The specific products needed for this method of oral care work *synergistically*, so that one step leads into the next—without the need to rinse with water between each step. The products are specific because each contributes a variety of benefits, and each works in harmony with the next step to help you achieve wonderful improvements in your mouth health, over and above any achieved by using one or other of the products *alone*. This also explains why adding or subtracting different products or generic substitutions will by necessity change the synergy of this system. Some people have used these exact products, but in the *wrong order*—and that misstep in protocol will also change the outcome. We know that any alteration in the sequence of cooking, together with use of different products or techniques, can completely affect recipe outcomes. The same principle applies here.

Sequencing

The length of time that you use the final rinses is somewhat flexible, but the method—or *sequencing*—of rinsing is vastly important and will help you to embrace just how easy it is to understand what each rinse does for you. Most people who time themselves say that daily application of this system takes less than five minutes, and it should be used twice each day (three times *maximum*) and *always* as the last dental care step that you take before you head off to sleep.

Success!

When the correct mouth biome balance has been achieved, you will notice progress and see the results you have been searching for. Within a few weeks, most people find that bad breath fades away, bleeding gums begin to heal, and any "fuzzy" feeling in your mouth will disappear as teeth start to feel clean, shiny, and smooth. And there it is, voilà—*success!* This is a great experience for everyone involved—in fact, I have heard several of my patients over the years describe this as achieving a feeling of having "happy teeth"—something that they had never contemplated as possible. What a wonderful thing it is to see dental problems *heal*.

ORAL CARE—A "NEW" APPROACH

Many people select a toothbrush or toothpaste by price-checking or by reading the promotional language on packages. For our best level of oral health, however, we need to apply a different set of criteria. We need to obtain and make consistent use of a high-quality toothbrush, coupled with a toothpaste that will help to heal cavities and reverse any areas of demineralization in the enamel. Many oral-care products are, frankly, quite useless. Some, in fact, can damage the oral environment and cause enamel to weaken—which leaves teeth more susceptible to decay. The worst thing any of us can do is to needlessly compromise the health of our teeth and/or gums.

There is an *art* to brushing your teeth, and a quantifiable *chemistry* that occurs between toothpaste and the enamel crystals that cover our teeth. A mouth rinse travels everywhere in the mouth—and although certain ones are helpful, others can damage teeth or upset the healthy bacteria in our mouth. In the United States, the products that I suggest can be sourced at local stores or online—and with relatively little expense.

Smoke and Mirrors vs. the Reality of Mouth Health

Many people believe—*incorrectly*—that optimal mouth health is achieved by straightening teeth into perfect alignment, and then whitening them artificially to create the "ultimate smile." You may like the way your teeth align, and you may be congratulated on your attractive white teeth, but it is the invisible *environmental* health of your mouth that is the control switch that determines the health of your teeth and gums—and how long you will keep them. If you ignore this measure of health and opt instead to cosmetically adjust your pearly whites through artificial methods, you can easily end up with a mouth in distress. These fixes are a temporary dental distraction from the disease and bacterial imbalances that are often lurking silently in a mouth, waiting for the moment to initiate recession, sensitivity, or other problems—perhaps at a time of stress or illness, during pregnancy, or in the later years of life, when these problems may cause chaos at shocking speed.

Today, we know the impact of a poor oral biome on a person's general health and how it contributes to the debilitating conditions of diabetes, arthritis, cardiovascular disease, and even premature birth—all while raising our risk for the horrible health outcomes of dementia, Alzheimer's, carotid artery blockage, and stroke among other maladies. Most people would never willingly ignore the slow progression of these health problems, but many people unwittingly allow this festering oral imbalance to exist in their mouths. Why does this happen? The big reason is because true mouth health is hidden behind a misleading curtain of superficial "tricks"—the smoke and mirrors of artificially whitened teeth, crowns, veneers, fake teeth, and implants.

It normally takes about ten years for the impact—or *symptoms*—of a mouth out of balance to become visible and be subsequently diagnosed by a dentist as cavities; fractured, weak, dead teeth; gum recession; or disease. The perception created by extraneous dental work that makes people look good can last for a time, often in a way that deludes us and pushes us further away from enjoying healthy teeth and gums. When you achieve environmental mouth health, your teeth, gums, tongue, saliva—your whole mouth, in fact—will become comfortable and disease-free, often within months.

This is why I want to explain the value of the Complete Mouth Care System™, which is a simple but strategic "do it yourself" method of mouth care that respectfully supports the natural processes of repair that occur every day. The changes you achieve are progressive and will be reflected by gradual improvements in the condition of your teeth and gums. Soon after you start this program, you will see changes—and your present and past dental history will become increasingly irrelevant. Do not focus on how many untreated cavities you have or worry that your gum problems are incurable or caused by age or family genes. When you use this system and balance your mouth health, it is a foregone conclusion that new cavities and gum disease will no longer occur. Environmental oral health cannot improve and deteriorate at the same time—it can only go in a forward or reverse direction, which is why you can be confident things are improving as soon as your mouth *feels* healthier.

STEP 1: PRE-BRUSHING RINSE

Many people have used mouth rinses as a quick way to "wash" their mouth, and basically clean up the smell of their teeth and/or breath. That may seem a logical action, but the difference here is that my system goes far beyond mouth washing, and into the realm of a treatment sequence designed to benefit your mouth and make it healthier.

Changes in Mouth Health

Dental visits should inform you about changes in your mouth health, and it is always encouraging to discover how much improvement you have achieved *between* dental visits—outcomes that are often far superior to those achieved by leaving your oral health in the hands of others. Unless you have an acute dental emergency, like a tooth abscess, I suggest that you use this system of care for at least three (3) to six (6) months before you begin any kind of dental treatment.

Certainly, not every cavity will completely heal with this home remedy—and yes, you may need a cleaning at some time, but this will be easier and more effective after you have used the system for six (6) months. Any filling or repair you need, maybe for some existing problem, will be easier if your enamel has hardened and when your mouth is healthy *before* the filling. This system will make your tooth stronger and less likely to fracture during treatment.

Another problem occurs if you already have a dead or dying tooth, because there is no way for this system to revive such a tooth. Treatment for a dead tooth is called a *root canal* and this is best performed by a specialist called an *endodontist*. A good root canal will allow you to save this tooth in your jaw and eliminate any spread of infection, which could cause damaging bone loss.

Even if you are someone who has suffered with hardened plaque under your gums, and your dentist has suggested a deep periodontal cleaning, or if he or she suggests skin grafting where you have lost gum tissues, all these periodontal treatments will heal faster and have improved outcomes if they are performed in a healthier mouth environment. This is why I encourage everyone to begin with the Complete Mouth Care System™—ideally, a few months prior to *any* treatment appointment.

The minute you feel or see small changes these should be a cause for hope—and for you to be encouraged. First, they illustrate your power to change your oral health; and secondly, it shows that what happened in the past—or the state of your teeth today—does not matter. Some changes that you notice may seem a little odd at first. Patches of decay can darken as they heal, and inactive plaque that is stuck to your teeth can create shadowy areas that sometimes make enamel look as if it is thinning or stained. These changes are annoying, but it is good to be forewarned and alerted to them, because such changes confirm progress and are good signals that your oral health is *improving*. There are several ways to manage and try to prevent staining from happening, and there are also several things you can do if you notice stains have already formed on your teeth.

Stains often happen within the first eight (8) to twelve (12) weeks of starting my system, and they are caused by the sudden improvement in your oral health, which can result in a shadowy superficial patch that becomes visible on tooth surfaces and sometimes between teeth. This kind of superficial staining is not harmful and is not permanent, but it signals that old plaque debris has deposited on your teeth—often in areas that are difficult to clean.

Plaque may have been stuck more firmly to tooth surfaces if your teeth were porous prior to starting this system, or if you had a sugar snacking habit. A professional cleaning can easily remove this surface color and leave your teeth shinier, and your underlying enamel health-ier and stronger than ever. If you want to try and remove this debris yourself, an effective idea is to sprinkle xylitol crystals on top of your toothpaste, at the toothpaste stage of the system. This slightly granular paste will offer more exfoliating power, and this may be sufficient to lift away the sticky plaque deposit. You will need to use a well-designed brush—preferably with flossing bristles, and never a sonic or soft brush, because removing this debris requires a good collection of densely resil-ient brush bristles.

Why a Pre-Brushing Rinse?

Perhaps you are standing in front of your bathroom sink, ready to brush your teeth. In this case, you may be surprised to learn that this system, or *process*, begins best with a mouth rinse. This first step dispenses with any possibility of causing abrasive tooth damage—a risk that can occur if tooth enamel is softened by acidic saliva or directly after a meal, snack, or drink. The stabilized chlorine-dioxide mouth rinse that I recommend—called **Closys** in the United States, and **Ultradex** in the United Kingdom—is a great way to prepare the mouth properly *prior* to brushing. This ultrasensitive formulation is unflavored and appears to be easier on the delicate gum tissues, which is helpful if your gums are sensitive or swollen.

A chlorine-dioxide rinse is most effective if it is unflavored. You may wonder if this colorless and tasteless liquid is working, but you need only wait a week or two to enjoy its initial effects. People are sometimes confused (particularly if they use pH testing paper to measure the acidity of their saliva or other liquids) because they may find that this particular rinse is acidic. This is not a problem because it is the way Closys *interacts* with saliva to form oxygen, which neutralizes mouth acids. The more acidic your saliva is, the more help you will need to neutralize it—and, consequently, more interaction will occur between your mouth and the rinse. So, I recommend this pre-brushing rinse to protect your teeth from abrasive brushing damage, to neutralize mouth acidity and help heal periodontal gum pockets around your teeth.

How Does It Work?

Closys will react with your saliva as it flows everywhere inside of your mouth—and it can even travel down the sides of teeth and into periodontal pockets, without the need for water-flossing or other similar devices. As this reaction occurs, oxygen is released. This process then disrupts the low-oxygen environments where harmful cavity- and gum-disease bacteria breed, which will benefit your gums and disrupt harmful bacteria in deep cavities and gum pockets. This is why Closys produces surprising results. Salt water may alkalize your mouth, but this would not help in the same way to combat cavities, pocketing, and periodontal gum disease. An additional benefit from Closys is that it addresses the bacteria that contribute to an unpleasant sulfur-smelling breath.

The "Exact One-Minute" Rule

The amount of Closys you use is not important, so only dispense enough rinse to be comfortably held in your mouth. On the other hand, this rinse must be accurately timed as it takes at least thirty (30) seconds for the rinse to interact with your saliva and travel into the gum pockets. You want to benefit from this released oxygen, so be sure to go beyond the traditional thirty (30) seconds that may be suggested and use Closys for exactly one exact minute of sixty (60) seconds *before* spitting it out to begin brushing.

Allow the liquid to bathe all your teeth, including back ones and areas where you suspect gum disease could be problematic—most often around molars, but sometimes also around your upper or lower front teeth. Be sure to tip your head calmly back and forth during the process for a full minute—so that all these areas are bathed fully with this mouthwash and then spit out and move on to Step 2, which is *brushing your teeth.*

STEP 2: BRUSHING YOUR TEETH

To keep our gums healthy on a consistent basis requires two things: An effective brushing technique; and the use of a bacterially clean and well-designed toothbrush. Another important element to a healthier mouth has much to do with *when* one starts to do things correctly—and when it comes to brushing one's teeth, the very best preventive move is to adopt a good brushing technique just as the first adult teeth erupt into the mouth during childhood. Fortunately, gum disease is not a risk for children under the age of five.

Gum problems can, however, begin to be initiated as new adult teeth enter a child's mouth soon thereafter around kindergarten age—and this is the time when parents should begin to pay closer attention, and when they should teach their children good brushing habits and how to do gum massage. It may take ten or more years for gum disease to become a full-blown mouth problem, but early gum massage can protect your child from problems by nipping this in the bud.

This is why the relevance of brushing teeth increases with a child's age, and the key for young children is mainly to establish an enjoyable habit every night before bed. The use of toothpaste for young children is optional—and we will discuss this further in Chapter Eight, where we will look more closely at methods of care for children of different ages. As adult teeth grow into the mouth, children can transition and begin to use a small amount of sodium fluoride toothpaste—the same kind that I recommend for adults. Most children will benefit from the entire system of care by their teen years when most, if not all, of their baby teeth will have been replaced by adult teeth. For children or adults with sensitive mouths, it is a good idea to use less paste and shorten the length of the two final rinses.

Next, let's take a look at *how* to successfully brush one's teeth—divided into the following parts, which you will next learn about in this chapter.

1. Brushing Strategy

Brushing is a vital part of this system, as it allows us to apply toothpaste to every tooth surface, to remove surface debris, *and* provide essential gum massage—all key elements in one's ongoing effort to keep the teeth and gums healthy.

Massaging your gums may be a new concept, as many people continue to believe that to brush one's teeth is merely to smear toothpaste over them. Most brushing habits among the general public have been found to be consistently inadequate, and serially unable to maintain or improve one's oral health. Since our gums first become susceptible to disease in our teenage years, it is ideal—for a successful long-term outcome—that we introduce children to the benefits of gum massage early in life. That said, it is *never* too late to begin your journey to better oral health—you just need to get *started*.

When it comes to cleaning tooth surfaces, the goal is to brush actively over every tooth surface *and* your gums—not only at the junction where the gums meet your teeth, but across all the surrounding gum areas. Your hygienist may be happy to help you learn how to brush better, so take your toothbrush with you at your next appointment—and request a personal demonstration (or learn from one of my online videos). Most children unfortunately believe they know how to brush their teeth by age four, and often they are never again instructed and therefore never learn the real goals and aims of effective brushing.

It is good to be a conscientious brusher. You should *always* think about what you are doing, as you work the brush around your mouth in an organized sequence. Be sure to brush the inner and outer surfaces of your teeth and gums. You should always target what you see as your more problematic areas *first*, even if you end up brushing over and around them twice. Gum massage also creates a steady movement of fluids in the gums—a naturally occurring assemblage of lymph liquids (which help to remove dead or unwanted cells from the mouth) and unwanted toxins that flow away in this liquid. This applied stimulation also brings a flow of blood to the gums and into the teeth that they support. The goal is to stimulate circulation and generate a wound-healing response in any area where your gums bleed, or where you have problems with gum disease or pocketing.

2. Toothbrush Selection

Select a toothbrush that can easily apply toothpaste throughout the mouth, but—more importantly—that will also help to keep your gums healthy. Standard brushes are designed for spreading toothpaste on to teeth, but you want to consider how well your toothbrush stimulates circulation in your gums. Ideally, look for so-called *flossing* bristles, which are designed specifically to help you access those areas between your teeth. It is good to ensure that the brush bristles will not damage your gums—to do so, look for a brush that is dense and outfitted with bristles of differing lengths.

You should have a brush that is hopefully not too soft, yet resilient enough to give your gums a good massage and remove debris from the tooth surfaces. You may have to buy a small selection of different brands and try them out yourself to get a better idea of what works best for you. There is no standardization of brush firmness—which creates difficulty for anyone who wants to determine if one brush is firmer than another. Simply put, the only way to know the best brush for you is to *try* a few. Some brushes may feel good for a few days, only to then rapidly become softer—and completely ineffective.

In an echo of the different bowls of porridge at the center of the classic fairy tale "Goldilocks and the Three Bears," your brush should not be too hard; too stiff; or too soft, since any of those qualities can render your brushing process ineffective—and therefore, not *just right*.

I do *not* recommend a technique known as *dry brushing*, which is when you massage your gums without any toothpaste or water on the brush, because this spartan approach to your teeth and gums can be too harsh. In fact, I suggest that if you feel that your gums or teeth are sensitive, then you should use warm water on your toothbrush before you apply paste. People who are lazy about brushing may find an electric brush more effective, but nothing beats a well-designed manual brush in the hands of someone who learns exactly how to use it.

Some people have developed a gag reflex that makes standard toothbrushes feel too big in their mouths. These individuals can often achieve success with *youth* brushes, provided that the bristles are as resilient as for adult brushes—just with a smaller brush head. Some people need longer handles or more angled heads, but generally look for a brush with plenty of bristles of differing lengths. No scientific evidence has yet shown that one type of toothbrush design is better than another, so perhaps try a few different ones to discover the one that allows you to brush most effectively.

Do your best to *not* select a brush for yourself that is too big, too small, or that has an ultra-long head. In general, the toothbrush head should be less than one inch in length with a handle that allows a firm grasp. The bristles must have rounded ends to avoid damaging the gums—the more bristles, the better. A brush with too few bristles will rarely be able to give your gums adequate massage, which is one of the secrets to generating gum growth and the perfect way to maintain one's gum health.

3. How to Clean Your Toothbrush

In recent years, people have begun to realize the hazards of using old and infected toothbrushes—but reports still indicate that the average American does not know how to clean a toothbrush, and only replaces it once or twice a year. My suggestion is not definite because an answer has not yet been scientifically proven. Some say you should change a toothbrush after an illness, but it seems most sensible to me that one should start to use a new brush after a cleaning, a periodontal treatment of any kind—and *especially* after surgery such as a skin grafting, an extraction, or a new implant.

Besides this, people with no dental problems who have a healthy mouth may be able to use the same brush for a longer range of time. If you have *two* brushes, and they dry for twenty-four (24) hours between uses, then the replacement time may be extended. I consider six (6) to twelve (12) weeks to be a reasonable interval, if you are using two brushes and if you are an established student of my Complete Mouth Care System™. If, however, your brother—who has no interest whatsoever in oral health—is asking how often he should change his dirty brush, then "A new brush every month" is likely the most helpful timeline to suggest.

It is important to keep toothbrushes sanitary and clean, because if you use an infected toothbrush, you risk introducing aggressive bacteria that can aggravate cavity and gum problems in your mouth. Any bacteria in your mouth or on your gums are transferred to your toothbrush bristles in a single use—and repeated use of an infected brush could replant these bacteria into your mouth.

Be aware of hazards that exist around your toothbrush if/when you travel; live in different spaces; or journey away from home while on vacation. It may be good to take inexpensive brushes with you and throw them away every few days—or disinfect them very carefully—especially upon your return. You could experiment with something different, like a Miswak stick, for use amid travel or temporary lodging. Brushes that are stored damp or wet inside travel bags can swiftly become infected with the kinds of bacteria that pose periodontal disease hazards. Studies show that one of the best ways to clean a toothbrush is to allow the head of the brush to air-dry completely between uses, and this can take up to twenty-four (24) hours for a brush with dense bristles. Generally, it is best to store a toothbrush head-up, in a cup, so that the bristles can dry. Always avoid damp or wet conditions where mold or bacteria can grow on your brush; for example, under a cover or inside a plastic bag—particularly if you are using a hollow rechargeable, or *sonic*, toothbrush.

Brushes stored close to others may also experience a transfer of bacteria, which is important to consider if you have cavities or gum disease in your mouth. It is also a concern in schools, daycare, and college dorms, where infected brushes can be a vehicle of transfer for harmful germs from one mouth to another. Avoid sharing brushes whenever possible—and if you doubt the air quality in your bathroom, then consider storing your toothbrush near a sunny kitchen window instead.

4. Choice of Toothpaste

People end up in trouble if they regard toothpaste as a "one-stop shop" for all their dental needs. A good toothpaste should *strengthen* your teeth (and thus whiten them naturally), just as it provides enough cleaning power to remove surface and bacterial debris—without, of course, scraping away a tooth's surface or negatively changing the tooth's natural structure. Generally, I suggest you avoid pastes with the added ingredient *glycerin*.

This area of concern was first raised in the 1960s by a chemist called Gerald Judd, who suggested that glycerin or glycerol could attract plaque to a tooth surface and become a barrier to successful tooth mineralization. Dr. Judd created his own experiments, which led him to record that it took twenty-seven (27) rinses to remove the film of glycerin from teeth. It is interesting that glycerin is the mainstay, and even the primary ingredient, in many commercial toothpastes—and yet, this study has *still* never been repeated with a controlled trial.

In spite of the hyperbole often expressed in promotional

language, the promised benefits from so-called "miracle" toothpastes will *not*: cure your dental problems; eliminate tartar; safely stop tooth and/or gum sensitivity; or naturally whiten your smile safely, and for the long-term. They *may* block porosity holes, kill bacteria, and strip away your mouth's protective barrier with chemicals that may *temporarily* appear to work—but what more commonly occurs is that these inferior pastes will instead sensitize your gums, causing the peeling and ulceration of your gums and the skin of your mouth.

Abrasive pastes can thin or weaken the enamel in your teeth. So, what you *really* need is a toothpaste that does not disrupt the mouth's bacterial balance or form a barrier layer on the outside of teeth, since this will prevent or delay the natural healing processes. The ideal toothpaste should safely clean all tooth surfaces, while it simultaneously speeds up the remineralization sequence that naturally strengthens tooth enamel.

If you have read this far, then you must certainly be asking yourself: What kind of toothpaste works best with this system? In answer to that question, I would recommend the original Crest Regular Cavity Protection toothpaste with no extras. This paste is 0.243% sodium fluoride and hydrated silica—both useful ingredients that fit perfectly into the sequence of my complete system of care. Never take your eye off the ingredient list of toothpaste and be sure to avoid *stannous fluoride*, a cheap tin/metal fluoride compound that kills oral bacteria and forms barrier plugs in tooth enamel. If you are using my recommended system but want to dilute the taste of the toothpaste, then sprinkle a quarter of a teaspoon (¼ tsp.) of xylitol crystals on top of the paste when applied to your brush, and you will find that it changes the overall *taste*—without changing the effects.

Benefits of a Good Toothpaste

For an adult, the amount of toothpaste you apply is not vitally important. However, for a child or young adult you should use only one (1) or at most two (2) small green pea-sized drops of paste on a damp brush head. If you find the taste of toothpaste too strong, simply reduce the amount of paste that you use. Target the surfaces of your front teeth, and then work around to other areas where you think you most need to remove plaque or food debris. If your hygienist has told you that your back teeth collect tartar, then this would be an area to target early in your brushing when you have the most toothpaste on your brush.

The kind of Crest toothpaste that I suggest (*see page 107*) cleans the surface of teeth without being too abrasive. It was formulated before the advent of the current whitening craze, but it *will* help to improve the color of your teeth by helping to mineralize the enamel surface—thus strengthening it, which makes it reflect light more completely. This paste also gives the enamel adequate protection from the relatively low acidity (pH level) of Listerine—the rinse that will now follow below as the next step of my system. This is why, at the end of brushing, you should spit out the toothpaste—but *do not* rinse the residual paste off your teeth with water, which would diminish the synergy of this system.

STEPS 3 AND 4: TWO FINAL RINSES— LISTERINE, FOLLOWED BY ACT

All liquid mouth rinses have their own unique chemical properties, and each has a different effect on our teeth, gums, and overall mouth health. The Complete Mouth Care System™ that I present here ends with a sequence of two final rinses—Listerine, and then the Anti-Cavity Treatment (ACT) fluoride rinse—which are used one after the other, a tag team of mouth rinses that do more than clean teeth. By using these *specific* rinses in the correct order listed above, they work in harmony to clean away harmful plaque bacteria (while sidestepping the mouth's good bacteria) but then they set the stage for natural tooth remineralization and gum support that will begin next.

This two-step ending is a robust way to stop cavities and help teeth strengthen and mineralize, while simultaneously promoting gum growth and setting up controls to stop plaque from forming— both above and below the gum line. Used in this tandem way, these mouth rinses enhance each other to leave your mouth feeling amazingly clean, and in time, they can deliver remarkable benefits. You may like to think of this duo in a similar way to the liquids used in skin care routines—where an astringent or toner will clean the skin, right before a protective moisturizer might be applied.

Listerine is used first, to rinse the toothpaste residue off your teeth while targeting immature plaque bacteria that may be floating in saliva. This rinse should be used by everyone—even those with a dry mouth—who have lost enamel or have sensitive or acid-damaged teeth. The Listerine rinse has effective cleaning power, but it is targeted to one kind of bacteria—and despite the claims of social media influencers among others, the formulations of Listerine that I recommend do not harm the mouth's microbial environment in any way. It is acidic, but this allows for a unique interaction with the final ACT rinse that is going to be used next. This duo creates a far more powerful mineralizing effect for teeth than simply using a fluoride rinse on its own. When this specific combination of two rinses is used in this sequence twice a day, they achieve a more complete and effective mineralization than any of the results achieved by using even strong prescription toothpastes, rinses, or fluoride varnishes.

Listerine—Effective Essential Oils

Listerine is a liquid that is scientifically classified as an *essential oil* mouthwash. Many people are surprised to find that the active ingredients are oils of the eucalyptus plant, together with the naturally occurring compounds menthol—from the peppermint plant—and thymol, which is extracted from the herbs thyme and oregano. The amount of ethyl alcohol in Listerine is 21.6%, and this is used to dissolve the oils into the mouthwash formulation. Studies by the American Dental Association (ADA) and the National Cancer Institute (NCI) show that the aforementioned alcohol in Listerine is present at a completely safe level. In this situation, the alcohol will immediately be diluted by saliva and then it will be finally rinsed away by the non-alcohol rinse ACT—which follows next.

Another concern that has been raised is the possibility of bacteria developing a tolerance to Listerine after continuous use, but studies show that the essential oils in Listerine do not result in bacterial resistance of any kind. Today, Listerine competes with many alternative choices, but it has survived all manner of online myths and many unfounded fears. And so, I remain fully confident that Listerine and ACT warrant their reputation as safe, and in the method that I suggest, you will likely be amazed how quickly this effective combination of rinses can improve your tooth and gum health to help you avoid the toxicity of fillings or other consequences of mouth imbalance.

How Listerine Works

In 1931, Listerine was the first mouth rinse to receive the American Dental Association (ADA) formal seal of acceptance after several twenty-four (24) week studies proved that it was able to control a plaque-induced gum inflammation known as *gingivitis*. Recent testing in multiple studies has confirmed the effectiveness of Listerine and also supported the company's research that shows rinsing twice a day with Listerine is five (5) times more effective than flossing, particularly when it is used every twelve (12) hours—twice a day.

Thymol targets a few problematic bacteria, yeasts, and fungi in the mouth, and the eucalyptus oil helps to promote gum growth. Listerine's effect is very specific toward immature plaque-forming bacteria such as *Streptococcus mutans*. Thymol can dissolve their hard outer coating, and because Listerine is a liquid, it intermingles with any plaque bacteria that are floating in saliva. The eucalyptus in Listerine is effective at helping to sooth gum problems, and this oil has been studied for its ability to help regrow gum tissue.

Enjoy Listerine

When selecting from the modern array of flavor choices, look for the original Listerine formula or the Cool Mint formulation. At the same time, be careful to avoid any rinses that are advertised specifically for plaque control or whitening, since many of these contain added chemicals or zinc that can make your mouth feel uncomfortable and make your teeth more sensitive to temperature changes that occur at mealtimes when we eat and drink. Many people find the taste of Listerine spicy, and if this happens to you—do not power through the feeling, but simply use it for less time and spit it out as soon as you are feeling a warm sensation in your mouth. A quick rinse is not problematic, as you will derive benefits from even a second or two. Notice the time you can tolerate Listerine and never go beyond sixty (60) seconds.

If your mouth has been damaged by the use of artificial whitening products, peroxide, baking soda, or frequent dental cleanings, then you will likely experience trouble rinsing, and you may not be able to tolerate Listerine for more than a few seconds. As your mouth health improves—a consequence of all the other parts of this strategy—you will find that you gradually work up to the thirty (30) seconds that are recommended for most people. Adjust the final rinse time to match the Listerine time—and when this duration with Listerine extends, increase the time you rinse with the ACT to match. The volume of Listerine in your mouth is not important—just use enough of it so that it remains a comfortable (dare I say *enjoyable?*) experience for you.

Be sure, of course, that you do not rinse with any water between having toothpaste on your teeth and the start of this Listerine step in the system. This allows toothpaste residue both to mitigate the taste of the Listerine and to offer your teeth protection from this rinse's acidity while it is in your mouth. Everyone will have their own personal tolerance level, and never go beyond a comfortable time or after you register a spicy signal on your tongue from the Listerine. The goal is thirty (30) seconds, and never longer than sixty (60) seconds maximum, but if you are uncomfortable or your mouth feels too hot—spit out the Listerine and rinse immediately (even after a couple of seconds), and then move on to the final ACT rinse.

Never forget to rinse Listerine off your teeth or the acidity of this rinse will work against you, promoting plaque and allowing cavities to get larger. It is with the last of these rinses that we turn possible problems into the finale that will benefit your teeth and gums.

Dilute Fluoride—The Final Rinse

For shiny, strong, and healthy teeth, I recommend that you rinse with a low-concentration sodium fluoride finishing rinse like ACT to protect your teeth at the conclusion of this system. This is because sodium fluoride supports, speeds, and stimulates the natural process of rebuilding tooth enamel, commanding minerals from saliva to enter the tooth and reconfigure the enamel crystals to make them more perfect, which helps to create naturally stronger tooth enamel.

How ACT Works

Although I filter fluoride out of my drinking water (see the section on fluoridation in Chapter Four from Part One of this book for the reason *why*), I *am* a proponent of using a 0.05% sodium fluoride rinse called ACT (anti-cavity rinse) as part of this system of adult tooth care, twice daily and always right before sleeping. It is especially important if you have damaged or weak teeth, lack natural protection (dry mouth), or are middle-aged or even older (which places you at higher risk for dental disease and damage).

A fluoride rinse is completely different from the undesirable idea of drinking artificially fluoridated water. Rinsing with a dilute fluoride compound will be helpful because it allows teeth to strengthen, and the surface enamel to become smoother and more fully mineralized—which is very helpful if your teeth are sensitive, if parts have broken or fractured, or if you have cavities. A fluoride rinse will also help to build weak enamel back to its former strength, which can also improve tooth color—all achieved without consuming any fluoride as you would if you were drinking it in your water.

A fluoride rinse will *also* help anyone with silver or white fillings in their teeth, because the surrounding enamel often loses its strength, which shortens the lifespan of fillings. This rinse can help you avoid ongoing and expensive filling repairs, and the consequences of these that may involve exposure to mercury or plastic chemicals as the fillings are removed, or damage to the tooth nerves that often happens and leads to tooth death and the need for root canals, crowns, or even tooth extraction and implants.

The Benefits of ACT

The volume of this fluoride rinse is not important, but you *do* want to monitor the length of time it remains in contact with your teeth. If you keep both final rinses comfortably in your mouth for thirty (30) seconds each, this will jumpstart your teeth to mineralize in the upcoming hour—and that process will begin the minute you have finished cleaning your teeth. If you can only use Listerine for a few seconds, you may *also* want to limit the ACT rinse to a similar amount of time and gradually work up to a longer time with both rinses simultaneously.

Always spit out well after the final rinses, and then rest your mouth by not eating or drinking anything for at least an hour afterward. The longer you wait before eating and drinking—*after* using my system—the more benefit for your teeth and gums. If you can wait and avoid all food and drinks for an hour or more, this action will enhance the benefits of the Complete Mouth Care System™, because if we allow more time for natural healing, more healing will occur. (This is something we have discussed in earlier chapters.)

WHEN TO USE THE COMPLETE MOUTH CARE SYSTEM™

Use this system twice a day, and a maximum of three (3) times a day. The essential time to use this system is before you head to bed each day, so that the strengthened tooth surface condition will protect your teeth while you are sleeping. This is particularly important for anyone who has a dry mouth, and *especially* those who breathe through their mouth at night. The other time should be separated by about twelve

(12) hours from this session. If you can use the system after a meal—which I can tell you works *very* well—you can design the timing of this system to conveniently mesh with your daily routines.

The "Happy Teeth" Timeline

I like to encourage everyone to take selfie photos as part of how they document their own respective oral health journeys. This may be the only way you will remember how your teeth looked and felt when you began using this system. There are scientific timelines that have been documented in various studies. For example, we now know how xylitol can help promote good bacteria while it also eliminates the bad. We also know that it takes one (1) month to stop plaque from aggregating on tooth surfaces, yet six (6) months before plaque will completely stop landing on them. This means you must brush most carefully during these first six months, but don't be discouraged—with use of my timeline provided below, you will be provided with a steady and dependable path toward your very own set of "Happy Teeth."

7 to 14 Days: If you have poor oral health, you may see and feel rapid improvements as your gums stop bleeding and visible plaque no longer forms on your teeth. This is the time when you need to work hard and try to brush your gums and teeth more effectively. Consider the periodic purchase of new toothbrushes and focus on how to do gum massage consistently and *effectively*. This will help you to remove old plaque from tooth surfaces and help prevent the stains that form when gums bleed and inactive plaque gets stuck on the surfaces of teeth.

3 to 6 Months: This may be a good time to arrange a return visit to your dentist for a thorough professional cleaning—in particular, to remove the debris of dead plaque from your tooth surfaces. Ensure that you use the system immediately before the appointment, and restart with some xylitol at the end of your visit. Don't expect accolades yet, and maybe keep your thoughts quiet this time around. It will be during your *next* visit when you should expect to be congratulated and hear about the improvements you have always wanted to achieve.

6 to 12 months: You should now be able to appreciate the changes that have occurred in your oral health, and you should feel empowered knowing *you* have the power to protect and strengthen your teeth. You can relax finally and enjoy this new confidence about your oral health. Maybe this is a good time for a professional evaluation, or a time to take photos, test your mouth bacteria, and maintain records of your improvements, as a reference for yourself. At this point—six (6) to twelve (12) months—your saliva should be free of new plaque bacteria, and any stains you have been fighting should become progressively less of a problem.

CONCLUSION

So, who can *use* the Complete Mouth Care System™? I am happy to report that this system is of great benefit for adult teeth (even for people with a dry mouth or acidic saliva); for the elderly and young; and for those who may think their situation is too far gone to correct or remedy. Pregnancy is a difficult time for teeth, but this system will help maintain and improve oral health during these months as well. It's particularly recommended prior to braces and orthodontic work, or when you are in the process of aligning teeth with retainers—a time that can stress your gums and teeth and lead to recession and tooth sensitivity.

There may be special situations, or in hospital or community settings, when the use of this system is not practical. This is when the use of xylitol may be all you can do, or perhaps just the toothbrushing with a small amount of toothpaste, or some combination of this with xylitol after meals, together with ACT rinsing.

In the next chapter, we will speak about what I consider one of the very best things to happen to mouth care in the past one hundred years—*xylitol*.

7

$\mathcal{X}$ylitol—
The Most Powerful Friend
a Mouth Can Have

Men judge us by the success of our efforts.
God looks at the efforts themselves.

—CHARLOTTE BRONTE

S ome years ago, a retired dentist friend of mine asked me how I use home remedies to help people avoid cavities. He wanted the secret because his wife's teeth were, in his words, "falling apart." Here was a wonderful dentist, an expert in his field, who could not protect his own wife from the plaque problems that were destroying her mouth. I explained how xylitol, and my system of mouth care, work in harmony to clean and protect teeth. Within weeks, my colleague told me with great excitement about the positive effects on his wife's oral health that they had noticed.

These same remarkable outcomes have been repeated for decades, consistently serving to amaze people with the benefits they quickly feel—and see. They often cannot believe that something so simple, and *delicious*, could make such an effective difference in the state of their mouths. If you are searching for oral health changes like these, then perhaps it is time for you to know more about *xylitol*— and how it can become a pivotal part of your daily dental regimen.

Another "real life" story concerns three teenage brothers, each of whom almost wrecked their oral health one summer as they enjoyed a month-long family camping trip. Before their new school year started, these boys would come together to visit me for their scheduled checkups—and were shocked to discover just how many cavities had surfaced since their last appointments. They admitted that consistent tooth care had been neglected during the summer and that they had enjoyed soda and snacks every day. Summer heat, and active lifestyles, had placed these boys at increased risk for oral disease, and the older brother's seasonal allergy medications had *additionally* caused mouth dryness—thus, creating even more potential for cavities to form.

I could see in each teen's mouth that the central grooves of the molars in their upper and lower jaws had started to decay—an alarming total of twelve (12) cavities between them in total. Instead of merely filling these cavities, I presented this family with another option—to go home and make daily use of xylitol, along with my unique system of care, to control their plaque infections and rebuild the lost tooth structure in each of their mouths.

The most important part of that family's decision, of course, was their choice to *act*—to make use of xylitol in harmony with my prescribed Complete Mouth Care System™ (as I have outlined previously in Chapter Six). Changing the situation for these boys was vital, since cavities simply progress if they are left alone and ignored. The boys carefully followed my directions and came for follow-up visits to monitor their progress at the three-, six-, and twelve-month marks. All twelve of those boys' cavities healed naturally, and *never* required fillings.

Ready to learn more about this seemingly magical oral health aid? Let me explain more about how it works and what it is.

XYLITOL 101

Xylitol (pronounced ZY-lih-tol) is a delicious granular health sugar that was first recognized as being good for oral health in the late

1940s. There had been a decade of sugar shortages in Great Britain, and so xylitol became an alternative sweetener for all kinds of baking; for use in beverages; and as a replacement for table sugar in most households. Xylitol can be extracted from the wood of birch trees, and so it is not surprising that The Finnish Sugar Company, located in a country where birch forests are plentiful, was one of the first to commercially distribute xylitol to other countries.

In Scandinavia (Norway, Sweden, and Denmark, specifically), xylitol is found in many of their candies, and for over six decades, Finland has managed a public health program for preschool and elementary schools, offering xylitol dental gum during school hours, every day. Switzerland also has produced xylitol and promoted it for oral health, launching a certification program in 1982 for tooth-friendly candy made with xylitol that meets their special regulation standards. Travelers to China, Asia, Turkey, and Japan are usually surprised by the selection of xylitol gum and mints in these countries—and how it has been promoted there, in children's playgroups and nurseries, for decades.

By the mid-1950s, European dentists and doctors had noticed—amid this more generalized consumption of xylitol—that the oral health of these populations had improved, and children in this part of the world not only experienced fewer cavities but less ear infections. This was a period of time when the first scientific research studies began to look at *why* these changes had occurred, and if xylitol actually *did* promote health. The benefits of this ingredient were gradually confirmed in decades of study conducted across many countries around the world—from Estonia to South America, and from China to Japan.

Xylitol first arrived in the United States in the middle of the 1960s, when it was incorporated as an active ingredient in healthy chewing gum. At this time in this country, however, there was comparatively little interest in natural health products. This gum was flavored with licorice and remained rated as a poor competitor alongside the tastier, longer-lasting, but artificially sweetened gum that the American marketplace had created for less health—and larger profits.

Today, xylitol can be purchased in granular form as well as in: tooth-friendly candy, with many fun flavors; breath mints; tooth gels; mouth rinses; baby products; and nasal sprays. Thankfully, xylitol-based products are no longer found only in health stores—they can be purchased nationwide, in a great many progressive grocery stores alongside other organic and natural products, and online from a large number of outlets (including, of course, Amazon.com).

WHAT IS XYLITOL?

As mentioned, xylitol was first produced from the fibers of birch wood, but it can be derived from a variety of hardwood trees, and it is also present in many popular fruits—including strawberries, raspberries, plums, and blackberries—and fifteen (15) grams is even created daily by the human body as a product of our metabolism. While this natural sweetener is now produced in several other countries around the world, using new techniques and processes (including *fermentation*—a process that is similar to brewing beer), the extraction of xylitol remains sourced primarily from fibrous plant materials like hardwoods, corn husks, and oats.

Granular xylitol is a colorless white crystalline powder, that not only looks—but also *tastes*—almost exactly like sugar, with perhaps a slightly fruitier flavor. This is where similarities between sugar and xylitol end—and enormous differences begin. Consuming xylitol creates an almost opposite effect of sugar in the mouth—in addition to being tooth-friendly, its benefits gradually promote oral health over time. In similar opposition to sugar's deleterious effects, consider the following: The more frequently we consume small amounts of xylitol each day, the more benefits we can achieve for our oral health. Consistent and frequent use of xylitol can progressively change a plaque-diseased mouth into one that is healthy and disease-free, with visible and measurable results, over a period of six months. It has truly given me so much pleasure and satisfaction over the years to see how quickly my patients have been able to turn their dental health around—just by taking my advice . . . and, of course, by taking xylitol.

THE BENEFITS

Many xylitol studies in the 1970s were centered upon populations of pregnant women, a group of individuals at increased risk for gum disease and cavity problems. These studies showed that when a mother consumed a single piece of one hundred percent (100%) xylitol chewing gum six (6) times per day, this small amount of xylitol—equal to about six grams of xylitol—had the power to control cavity-forming bacteria in these mothers' mouths. Furthermore, this change impacted and controlled the spread of the cavity forming infection to the newborn babies who were followed for years and found at age six to have eighty-five percent (85%) fewer cavities than the control group of children in the study. A later study in 2022 conducted in the East African country of Malawi showed that two pieces of xylitol-infused chewing gum—consumed by thousands of high-risk pregnant mothers after lunch, and before sleeping at night—significantly reduced their overall chance of delivering a child prematurely.

These are the kinds of exciting studies that have illustrated the attributes of xylitol for prenatal and family health. Many other studies and clinical trials have shown the benefit of xylitol for cavity prevention in early childhood. Research conducted at the University of Washington Dental School by Peter Milgrom, DDS, indicated how much xylitol is necessary to achieve these effects and looked at the timeline of how plaque is gradually controlled over a period of six (6) months.

Meanwhile, Kauko K. Makinen, PhD—who has had an amazing career at the Universities of Washington, Michigan, and Turku in Finland—has led many studies and has shown how the frequency of xylitol use (even in tiny amounts) affects the rate of decay in children's teeth, and how regular use of small amounts at the end of meals can lessen the chance that a cavity will develop in a child's mouth. Consistent use of xylitol therefore appears to be one of the most effective ways to enjoy its protective dental benefits. The results you get depend on your personal discipline; but seeing improvement always makes this easier.

The *Truth* About Xylitol

There have been decades of studies on xylitol, showing its oral health benefits and how it also provides a variety of positive health effects. Throughout this chapter thus far, we have discussed how xylitol can interrupt the family transmission of plaque bacteria; how it can help to control tooth decay in children and adults; and how it has been shown to reduce the incidence of premature birth for pregnant mothers. It is therefore useful to consider what was discovered about xylitol according to the following timetable—and be aware that all cited studies and research below reflect a one-hundred percent (100%) level of xylitol:

● In 2019, the Society for Global Health and Nutrition reviewed the attributes of xylitol beyond mouth health, by exploring the positive health impact of xylitol on the respiratory system for nasal, throat, eat, and sinus health. This article also documented how xylitol can help increase bone strength and reduce body inflammation—positive effects that help to prevent cardiovascular events, arthritis, and diabetes. In other studies xylitol was shown to support immune health, and even more remarkable were the results of xylitol for controlling a variety of viral and bacterial infections (especially the influenza virus, when xylitol was combined with red ginseng). Xylitol was also shown to be a benefit for weight management, and have beneficial effects on metabolic health, with an ability to increase a feeling of satiety after eating.

● In 2020, more exciting results emerged from a Japanese study reported in the scientific journal *Chemico-Biological Interactions* that xylitol showed some anti-cancer effects, and how a chemotherapeutic strategy combined with xylitol might improve the outcomes for patients facing cancer.

● Then by 2022, a *meta-analysis*—which is defined as the scientifically deep and complete review of past studies—was conducted to evaluate the effectiveness of xylitol for the prevention of *dental caries* (tooth decay). The results were published in the *Journal of the International Society of Preventive and Community Dentistry*, and they showed—once again—that one hundred percent (100%) xylitol is most effective in preventing tooth decay when used three (3) to five (5) times a day, and when the total dose is between five (5) to ten (10) grams of xylitol daily. The conclusion of this analysis was that xylitol should be part of our overall oral health strategy for children and adults.

This is why it was so shocking in June 2024 to read media articles that reported how xylitol could increase our risk for cardiovascular events. The study at the center of this coverage, funded by private equity groups, was hard to access as it was initially behind a paywall, and this inconvenience was compounded by extremely misleading media reports. The interested individuals who read the study from the source were able to dispute these inaccurate media articles and explain that the study only has relevance—and any possibility for concern—in elderly individuals who are suffering from health conditions that included diabetes; high blood pressure; and cardiovascular disease if they consume extremely large amounts of xylitol as a drink after fasting.

In the study, there were no control groups taking smaller amounts, which could have helped ensure the efficacy of the results—and the oral health, diet, and smoking statuses of these subjects was not reported. Furthermore, the group of ten (10) subjects in this study were given an unusually large dose of xylitol—thirty (30) grams, in fact—as a drink, immediately after fasting. None of the study group suffered any adverse clinical reaction from this drink—but their blood was tested, and researchers found a small elevation that averaged six percent (6%) in the concentration of certain metabolites in their blood samples. Anyone who is concerned by this statistic should consider that these percentages can be elevated by one to two hundred percent (100–200%) in patients who smoke cigarettes.

The report from the Cleveland Clinic, which was the study center, specifically stated that this particular study had no relevance to the insignificant amounts of xylitol recommended for oral health. This fact was **never** mentioned by the media—instead, many outlets put images of chewing gum, even *toothpaste*, as an attraction alongside their scary headlines. Our body makes fifteen (15) grams of xylitol each day through the processes of metabolism, but it is quickly and completely metabolized, usually clearing away to baseline within an hour—and *never* creating a buildup of xylitol in our body. It is unfortunate that media reportage remains so focused on creating unnecessary fear by disseminating inaccurate information.

Looking instead at statistics from countries where it has been consumed commonly for over sixty years, it appears that even the elderly should feel confident to follow sensible guidelines for the use of xylitol —perhaps aiming for five (5) to ten (10) grams of xylitol per day and spacing this consumption at the end of meals ideally with an hour afterward when they do not eat or drink.

HOW MUCH SHOULD YOU USE?

The amount of xylitol required to protect the growing teeth of infants and young children is less-than-half a teaspoon per day (2–3 grams). For adults, the ideal amount is between one and two teaspoons daily (5–10 grams). In each scenario described above, the amount of xylitol needs to make direct contact with teeth frequently each day, but the duration of interaction can be short. This means we have a choice to either brush our teeth with xylitol (by sprinkling the granular xylitol crystals on a damp toothbrush) or to instead enjoy xylitol as mints or chewing gum at the end of meals consumed during the day.

Xylitol loses some of its benefits when the crystals are dissolved in water, but this application may be useful to brush or clean the teeth of an infant or debilitated patient of *any* age. In every case, xylitol's benefits are multiplied when its frequency of use is increased, and when this xylitol exposure is followed by a period of *mouth resting,* which is any time when saliva in the mouth is allowed to remain without any change in dilution. Put more simply, it is a time of "no eating or drinking" whenever xylitol is consumed.

In 2006, the aforementioned Dr. Milgrom showed that adults need at least three (3) grams of xylitol per day to create positive oral health changes—while less than this may not create any visible oral health changes, such as a reduction in plaque on teeth or improved gum health. This is why it is suggested that one (1) to two (2) grams of xylitol be consumed at the conclusion of every meal or snack, to create an ideal frequency of ingestion about five (5) to six (6) times per day. When the amount of xylitol consumed daily is *above* ten (10) grams, any effects in the mouth will plateau—meaning that it does not appear to produce any additional benefit to one's oral health.

WHY XYLITOL? MY STORY.

My personal passion for xylitol grew to the point of starting a xylitol mint and gum company in the 1990s. I had moved from the UK to live in America but during this transition I had to wait to take the necessary courses and for my dental license to be approved. This was an era prior to Starbucks, and I was looking for a cup of cappuccino, so I decided to open a coffee shop in Rochester, New York.

The first cafe was very small, but it quickly grew into a sizable operation with over forty employees. I was aware that many of these employees had poor oral health and inadequate funds for the dental treatments they required, so I naturally introduced them to the benefits of xylitol and made a peppermint flavored mint that we dispensed from a gum-ball dispensing machine at the back of the restaurant. The restaurant had a large bakery, and so it was common for employees to snack on cookies, cake, and, of course, coffee and soda. Before serving tables, the staff would regularly freshen their breath with a sugary breath mint—the "icing on the cake" for placing them at risk for horrible cavities and dental problems. The new breath mint I made was formulated with one hundred percent (100%) xylitol—and *flavored* with peppermint.

Something to Think About

It is important to note that xylitol is an expensive ingredient, which is why many commercially available xylitol products contain percentages of xylitol so low that they will not work effectively in my system of mouth care. This is why it is so crucial to only select products that are made with one hundred percent (100%) xylitol.

So, the new breath mints that I had created were embraced by my staff, and soon became a daily routine in their lives—this simple substitution for the sugary mints they were eating at their coffee breaks seemed to have done the trick. Of course, they continued to enjoy sweet treats, coffee, and some even smoked cigarettes—but now, by ending their coffee break with xylitol, they suddenly saw stunning improvements in their dental health.

This was also a time when I was working as Faculty at the University of Rochester, under the guidance of a professor who had been involved in the xylitol studies of the 1970s. I suggested that we should repeat these studies, which had been conducted in South America, to prove the long-term effects of xylitol. As the director of the outpatient pediatric clinic at the Eastman Dental Center during this same period, I believed that we could study how xylitol had the power to interrupt the transmission of cavity bacteria from mothers to their babies. Furthermore, I maintained that we could *then* use this research opportunity to help pregnant women at the nearby maternity centers headquartered in Rochester, New York's Strong Hospital.

Using the normal protocol necessary prior to starting any research, I tried to obtain funding for this study, but with no positive response or show of interest from the funding authorities. I was told, in no uncertain terms, that there was no money for a project that would not benefit dentistry or the university. Mystified (and, frankly, *shocked*) by this total lack of interest in finding a cure for cavities, I decided—there and then—to further pursue the results of my discovery on my *own*. And so, I soon resigned from my position at the university and drew out my retirement savings to start my own xylitol company and teach the public directly about the best ways to use xylitol.

As anyone with their own business knows, starting something new is difficult. However, I ran into a lot of wonderful people—and a good amount of *luck*—that proved invaluable to me on this journey. As I pointed out earlier in this chapter, the mints that I had made for my restaurant staff were made with xylitol (pronounced aloud as if the word begins with the letter "Z"). The waiters merged this "Z" with my name "Ellie," and then simply added an "s"—thus giving an informal "in-house" name to those little mints of mine, a catchy term that I would soon elect to use as my new company's name . . . **Zellie's.**

Zellie's was incorporated in 2004 and has grown steadily in production and distribution over the years. This business has given me a wonderful platform from which to continue teaching the science of oral health—but I am no longer confined to medical and dental students alone. Instead, I have elected always to educate *anyone* who is interested, and I have continued to do so with: presentations in libraries, grocery stores tasting tables, at various gatherings in hotel ballrooms and events, in groups; through the production of an online video course; and, finally, on a near-constant basis through all manner of social media.

To the immense frustration of anyone who cares about their teeth, there *still* seems to be a hiatus in research around prevention of dental disease—and a consistent failure to direct the knowledge and resources that we have achieved at this point to eliminate this ongoing and burdensome health issue. Considering all that we now know, it seems all but certain that history will be especially harsh toward the profession of dentistry if they do not soon start to accept this new paradigm of patient empowerment—and willingly embrace a different and more patient-centered approach to oral care.

HOW TO USE XYLITOL

For adults to fully maximize the benefits of using xylitol, the following two basic steps are ideal:

1. Place one-eighth of a teaspoon ($\frac{1}{8}$ tsp.) of freestanding granular xylitol crystals directly into your mouth or purchase a form of xylitol that has been either compressed into a mint—chewing gum is another suitable vehicle that can be sweetened with xylitol—to then deliver a gram of xylitol directly into the mouth at the end of meals. Most mints contain a half-gram of xylitol, so two mints—or one piece of one hundred percent (100%) xylitol chewing gum—will provide a gram of xylitol at the conclusion of meals and after snacks.

As the xylitol dissolves in your mouth, it should be enjoyed for its taste and then swallowed—like any other candy or mint. Mints can be sucked or crunched up, and *then* swallowed. If you use gum instead, do not chew it for longer than ten minutes—by which time

127

KISS YOUR DENTIST GOODBYE

the sweet taste should be gone. Longer gum chewing will bring a different kind of digestive saliva into the mouth, which will dilute and wash away the xylitol-stimulated saliva that is most useful for healing the gums and teeth.

2. It is ideal immediately after each xylitol exposure to have a period when you do not eat or drink for *at least an hour*—something that I call *mouth resting*. This allows saliva with xylitol dissolved in it to interact with the mouth and teeth, and for xylitol to work in what is called a *prebiotic* capacity, which serves to nurture the mouth's population of good bacteria.

Be forewarned, though, that if you snack on xylitol too frequently (without giving the mouth adequate resting time between), you may actually *lessen* its positive effects. Constant snacking on xylitol or trying to orchestrate a way to keep it in your mouth for longer periods (as opposed to just enjoying and swallowing it) may cause areas of exposed root dentin to *feel* temporary sensitivity. This does not damage your teeth or gums, but it is an unnecessary and painful sensation that is more probable if you have thin enamel, exposed root areas from gum recession, or an unfilled cavity in your mouth.

Something to Think About

Be aware that when it comes to the maintenance of a healthy microbiome in the mouth, the use of *probiotics*—or living strains of good bacteria—will not work in the same way as they function in the digestive tract. It is important to distinguish carefully between *digestive* and *oral* probiotics, since research shows it is very difficult to introduce any new strains of bacteria into the oral microbiome. The best approach is to support oral bacteria by giving them time to interact with saliva periodically throughout the day, and support saliva health by a good diet that promotes digestive health.

Xylitol's beneficial effect happens because of its ability to pull saliva into the mouth—a process known as a *hygroscopic pull*. The saliva that is thus attracted into the mouth is the magical liquid that will help to heal your teeth and gums, provided we allow time for this particular interaction to occur. Success with xylitol is achieved most effectively when you stop overthinking the "dental" nature of xylitol—and just enjoy the taste and fun of eating it!

Many foods and supplements improve digestive health by nurturing healthy digestive bacteria, and there are so-called *digestive prebiotics*—an assortment of non-digestible fibers found in various vegetables, fruits, and whole grains—that help to *feed* these good bacteria in our digestive tract. It is wonderful to know that xylitol functions as this kind of fiber and works as a prebiotic to support specific gut bacteria that produce a health-promoting compound (known as a short-chain fatty acid called *butyrate*).

New research indicates that butyrate may have an impact on blood glucose regulation, and consequently a neuroprotective effect on our brain. Butyrate also helps to strengthen the gut's barrier lining, which can aid in reducing the risk of deteriorative digestive conditions. When the gut lining is damaged, this allows substance to leak from the inside of the gut and migrate to the *outside*. This means that substances and bacteria that should rightfully remain inside the gut walls instead begin to "leak" elsewhere throughout the body, where they can initiate a severe inflammatory response that can cause many more unpleasant symptoms for the patient. These problems occur because there is excessive *intestinal permeability* (known more popularly as "leaky gut"), and the most common trigger for this—according to the Cleveland Clinic—is the chronic overuse of antibiotics, alcoholic beverages, and/or popular over-the-counter non-steroidal anti-inflammatory drugs (NSAIDs) like aspirin and ibuprofen.

After Antibiotics

Another opportunity for xylitol to improve oral health occurs during and after any course of antibiotics that you may have had prescribed for you. Antibiotics are used for all kinds of bacterial infections and each course will exert a widespread effect on the body's entire bacterial population. No matter the reason for an antibiotic prescription, the effect will simultaneously reach and potentially disable bacteria everywhere in your body to some degree—often with the greatest impact on the mouth and digestive bacteria. This is why, following a course of antibiotics, we can jump on this and see it as an opportunity to *refresh* our digestive and oral bacteria and *improve* them.

Digestive or "immune health" probiotics (defined earlier in this chapter) may be useful following a course of antibiotics, but I suggest you focus on eating foods that are supportive of your immune health and high in fiber at the same time. This would be foods like mushrooms, garlic, onions, green leafy vegetables, avocado, fruits, and salad greens for a start. The goal is to support your digestive health and, in this way, influence and improve the uptake of minerals from all the foods you are consuming. These minerals will circulate around your body and find their way into your saliva liquids, which then helps to support your oral health. Taking an oral probiotic (as opposed to a digestive probiotic) would be less important—and at the present time, there are not enough studies to indicate specific long-term benefits from these expensive supplements.

Ear, Nose, and Throat Infections

At first glance people are surprised by the link between mouth bacteria and ear, nose, and sinus infections. You will recall that in Chapter Two we looked at the anatomy of the throat; how it connects the nasal passages to the mouth; and how tubes run from the back of the throat and into our ears. *Otitis media* is an infection inside these ear tubes, and children between the ages of six (6) months and two (2) years old are frequently affected because, at this age, these tubes lie horizontally, which allows saliva to access the entrance of these tubes.

The American Academy of Pediatrics (AAP) reported in 2000 that doctors wrote more than 800 prescriptions for every thousand children they treated for ear infections. The use of antibiotics can develop drug-resistant bacteria and upset the child's digestive health early in life. Children with recurrent ear infections are at higher risk for learning problems, not to mention the pain and suffering these children and their families experience. By reducing sticky plaque bacteria in the mouth and nasal passages with xylitol, this can limit the potential for sticky bacteria to gain access to these ear tubes. Studies show that young children using xylitol *preventively* in the form of xylitol mints or as a xylitol nasal spray experienced forty-two percent (42%) fewer ear infections, especially children prone to respiratory problems.

BAKING WITH XYLITOL

In the year 2000, I was asked to speak at a hygiene conference in Syracuse, New York. To introduce these hygienists to the wonders of xylitol, I provided coffee and brownies to them all. I explained the oral and general health benefits of xylitol and then shared the xylitol treats with my intrigued and excited audience. Many of those first converts remain enthusiastic proponents of xylitol today.

Karen Edwards was the xylitol enthusiast who introduced to me the idea of baking with xylitol. Karen is a nutritionist who wrote a book in 2003 titled *Sweeten Your Life the Xylitol Way*. She has baked with xylitol for years and has developed a line of dessert sauces under a brand called Karen's Kitchen, Inc. The main problem with using xylitol for cooking is that if people suddenly eat large quantities of xylitol—to eliminate sugar from their diet—they can notice a laxative effect at first, because xylitol is digested as fiber in the gut.

The best advice is to first experience xylitol *gradually*, especially if you are replacing sugar in your diet. Personally, I believe there are many healthy options for sweetening foods, including maple syrup, honey, stevia, raw cane, allulose, monk fruit, and coconut sugars. For myself, I prefer to enjoy lots of different sugars in cooking and use xylitol as a tooth-friendly *ending* to meals. Granular xylitol is found in the baking section of most health food stores, in bulk bags or teaspoon-size packs.

Warning—*Not* for Dogs!

The only warning I would give you about xylitol is that it should never be given to pets—and dogs, in particular. Keep xylitol candies, mints, gum, and other products out of the reach of pets. There are many delicious human foods that are not good for dogs—grapes, chocolate, raisins, and avocado—to name a few, and xylitol is yet another of these foods.

SWEET CONFUSION

Most people who know the difference between natural and artificial are quite confused in the world of sugar alternatives. Not all sugar replacements are artificial and there are many naturally-occurring low-calorie sugar alternatives derived from plants, and fruits like raisins and figs—products like stevia, monk fruit, and allulose. Some of these are intensely sweet, whereas others closely resemble the texture and taste of sucrose sugar. Combining stevia powder with monk fruit, for example, makes the intensely sweet stevia more manageable when mixed with the less sweet and bulkier monk fruit sugar.

Be warned that naturally derived sugar alternatives can also be mixed with one or more less expensive *artificial sweeteners*—products that often have alluring, industry-created names like Truvia, Ever-Sweet, Splenda, Sweet 'n Low, or Equal. Artificial sweeteners have been promoted in the United States for decades, allowing consumers to assume they are safe, but in the world of sweeteners, names and appearances are deceptive.

There is also a confusing classification of products called *sugar alcohols*. Xylitol lives within this group although it should really be set apart because it has a different chemical structure from other sugar alcohols. None of these sugar alcohols has any likeness to the liquid we call "alcohol;" the name is a chemical description of their molecular structure. Xylitol, for example, is a *pentose* or five-carbon molecular structure. All other sugar alcohols have a *six*-carbon structure which is, in fact, similar to the six-carbon structure of sucrose sugar.

Unfortunately, many dentists are equally confused by all these different sugars and classifications, even though studies show there are big differences in oral health impact between chewing xylitol gum and chewing gum sweetened with the carbohydrate compound called *sorbitol*. Xylitol is expensive and so many commercial gums and candies mix it with cheaper variants—often *sorbitol*, or the sugar alcohols *mannitol* or *maltitol*. Frequent consumption of sorbitol can, however—after several grams have been ingested—start to feed plaque and cause stomach cramps and digestive discomfort. This is why there is a big difference between xylitol and sorbitol and why it is important to *never give sorbitol to children under the age of three*, or to adults at risk for acid reflux.

The body utilizes xylitol in a way that is in total contrast to refined *sucrose* (sugar), and different from the sweetener *sorbitol* mentioned above. A small amount of pure xylitol each day can play an important part in helping infants and young children grow up with healthy teeth—and it is *equally* useful for healthy aging. Studies show xylitol's positive effects on the digestive microbiome, promoting communities of bacteria that create a short chain fatty acid known as *butyrate*, a compound that improves the health of our digestive tract lining to allow better absorption of minerals from the foods we eat. The health of our digestion often deteriorates with age; compromises our immune system; and opens the door to new, or more severe, chronic health conditions, which can become progressively more debilitating in later life—conditions such as diabetes, arthritis, cognitive decline, cardiovascular events, and even loss of bone density.

CONCLUSION

It seems an understatement to declare xylitol a revolutionary and healthful product. Using xylitol is not only a pioneering idea, but it is the first natural product poised to radically—and *wonderfully*—disrupt dentistry's old understanding of cavities and plaque. Initially, medicine had no understanding of germs—for thousands of years, doctors believed that disease was caused by imbalances in four body liquids called *humors*. Medical treatments from this era appear cruel and barbaric when we think about how illness is treated today, but physicians were helping patients in the only way they knew at that time. Dentists have tried to follow in the tailwinds of medicine, but they have been unable to find pharmaceuticals to stop cavities or gum disease. This is why dentistry clings to what it sees as its only apparent option: tooth amputation (drilling), prosthetic replacement (fillings), and mechanical dental cleanings.

Now is the time for a major shift in the way we care for our teeth; for dentistry to embrace healthy mouth bacteria as allies for oral health and to more deeply question its approach to cavities and gum disease. This new vision empowers every individual to take charge of their personal oral health, and xylitol becomes a precious resource in this endeavor. I do not believe xylitol is a miracle health panacea. However, if we work to develop healthy habits, offer our body adequate periods of rest and regeneration, and work toward a diet that includes a wider diversity of *healthy* foods, then I am convinced xylitol can be a solid partner in all of our oral health efforts.

In the next chapter, we are going to explore how xylitol and my Complete Mouth Care System™ can provide far-reaching and potentially surprising benefits to anyone prepared to test the idea that cavities and gum disease are not only controllable, but even reversible.

8

---

*W*hen Your Mouth Goes South—How to Stop High-Risk Dental Issues

We delight in the beauty of the butterfly
but rarely admit the changes it has gone
through to achieve that beauty.

—MARGUERITE ANNIE JOHNSON (MAYA ANGELOU),
PIONEERING AMERICAN POET

It's human nature to want a "quick fix" for our problems. In the dental world, there has remained—since the late 1800s, in fact—the idea that dentists provide a quick fix as they drill and fill teeth. Originally, fillings had seemed to be a great alternative to tooth extractions. We now understand, however, that each of us has the power to prevent tooth damage, reverse early cavities, and avoid unnecessary dental drilling, fillings, and other treatments.

If you are someone who has already experienced what has seemed like a never-ending history of dental problems, failed procedures, and extreme dental expense, then you know firsthand how frustrating it is to hear that cavities can be prevented and even reversed . . . while you have been seemingly excluded from these solutions. The first thing to know is that it is never too late to gain control of your mouth health, and this chapter is going to further explain how it can work for you (with the use of xylitol, and the additional benefits delivered by my Complete Mouth Health System™).

"PERFECT STORM" DENTAL CHAOS

When it comes to oral health woes, the reality is that dental problems are created by a confusing mix of circumstances that function as a kind of "perfect storm" environment around our teeth. Despite so many advancements in the world arena when it comes to new technology and medical research, dentistry still has never found a solution to combat the less-than-ideal conditions that cause tooth and gum damage—and so it continues to focus on ways to repair the damage and dissipate any accompanying pain and discomfort.

There is only one way to stop these ongoing issues, and that is to address the underlying *cause* of dental problems. Since there is no single product that can remedy a combination of perfect storm conditions, dentistry considers these problems to generally be *genetic* in nature—and, therefore, all the disease and damage lies outside, and *beyond*, our control.

The truth is that, with the use of my Complete Mouth Care System™ and the kind of consistent xylitol-based strategies first discussed in Chapter Seven, you can forge a path out of all this dental health chaos. Many of the solutions for dental problems that have been proposed by traditional dentistry create a new cascade of unexpected consequences. This is the dental dance you may have personally experienced—one step forward, three steps back. A dentist fills a cavity in your tooth, but then the enamel cracks . . . a gap opens up between the filling and the enamel . . . liquids and infection travel under the filling . . . and now the filling fragments and fails . . . and the cavity is so deep it has killed the nerve, so now you have a dead tooth that needs a root canal . . . then a crown . . . an extraction . . . perhaps then an *implant*. Then another tooth begins to experience the same story—one tooth after another. Sound like a nightmare to you? You're right, it *is*!

All those who have experienced this sequence of events will surely now be nodding their heads, relieved and comfortable in the knowledge that I understand what they have suffered. On the other hand, I realize there will be others who think this story is just alarmist. The fact is that if you have a dry mouth, or are someone with acidic saliva, then this is likely an exact replay of your dental misery—even if you are someone who has flossed and brushed religiously and gone to every dental cleaning. Why does this only happen to certain people? Of course, you could believe it is your fate or that you have inherited these problems—but this is *untrue*. The solution is entirely within your reach, and it lies in balancing your mouth health with the strategies I recommend.

Over the years, dentistry has looked for solutions and ended up being compulsively attracted to a multitude of "shiny new things." This slew of new products and ideas became popular recommendations in dental offices for a while—that is, until frustration and disappointment inevitably arose. Do you remember fluoride gels, remineralizing pastes, or maybe the *charcoal* method? Charcoal, it turns out, became the "darling" of the dental world around 2018 as people began to search for more "natural" ingredients in their oral care products. There was never any evidence of an advantage from using charcoal, but the claims of marketers created its fleeting fame. In the early 2000s, even toothbrush filaments were coated with it; black toothpaste was made with it; and influencers on social media seemed certain that charcoal was the best "way" to whiter teeth.

In 2001, a study published in the *Journal of Dental Research*, and another in the *International Journal of Dental Hygiene* looked at the abrasiveness and whitening effect of charcoal-containing toothpaste. This was a time when people began to complain that charcoal was making their teeth far more sensitive to changes in temperature, and that their tooth enamel was wearing away. The abrasiveness of the toothpastes on enamel and dentin was studied and found to range broadly. Finally, after these studies the American Dental Association (ADA) warned of the abrasive nature of charcoal and the fact that toothpaste is more effective when it contains a little fluoride. As one product exits the stage, the next enters in an ongoing performance to introduce the *next* acclaimed "shiny new thing." Some of us view this as a cruel and senseless game of dental hijinks that may give you hope for a while but will never actually provide a solution that stops the painful, damaging, and *expensive* problems of cavities and gum disease.

Xylitol as "Shiny New" Outlier

So, why hasn't xylitol ever been introduced as a "shiny new" dental solution? The reason may be that xylitol is not new and does not offer a simple solution to dental problems. Xylitol is a unique tool that must be used in a specific way so that it allows the mouth to heal itself. It requires that we are consistent in our daily use and that we have a diet and habits to support its actions. There is no way to promote xylitol as a dental "miracle" product—and it does not perform as effectively in the form of a toothpaste or mouth rinse as it does when it is consumed as an after-meal candy or gum.

This message may have been too difficult in past years for dentistry and was perhaps seen as too complex a concept for dental marketing. A smattering of television advertisements from the 1990s can be found on YouTube, in which xylitol was in fact promoted as being better than a toothbrush and an accepted routine for adults and kids to enjoy before going to bed at night. You can even find advertisements for xylitol toothpaste made by the Colgate-Palmolive corporation during this period.

The dental industry itself was, for a moment, frustrated by its lack of control over cavities and gum disease. Any dentist in the early 2000s who was interested to solve the increasing and serious problem of decayed teeth in America may have participated in an idea proposed by the American Dental Association (ADA). We were actively encouraged to become accredited "evidence-based champions"—to learn more about statistics and how to evaluate the quality of research, and to become more fully aware of the system or processes with which to correctly assess published studies.

Following participation in this course, we were then invited to attend an evidence-based conference in Bethesda, Maryland, hosted by the National Institute of Dental and Craniofacial Research. This professional gathering was organized to closely examine groups of studies and, with the help of top scientists, determine from the best evidence how dentists should help prevent and manage cavities and tooth decay.

I can still recall the shock that there was really no evidence to support brushing, flossing, or even fluoride supplementation. I also remember just how strongly xylitol emerged as the biggest topic of enthused conversation during that conference, and it was immediately introduced by the US military to help deployed soldiers ward off cavities in a program called "Look for Xylitol First." Dr. Catherine Hayes, an associate professor in the department of Oral Health Policy and Epidemiology at Harvard University, ended the conference with her comment that it could be perceived as unethical to deprive people of the benefits of xylitol as it can "significantly decrease the incidence of dental caries."

WHAT ABOUT TOOTH SENSITIVITY?

Perhaps you are someone who is plagued by tooth sensitivity, an uncomfortable sensation in your mouth that is a definite cry for help—from your *teeth*. Trust me, you do not want to silence this alert by using sensitive or mineralizing pastes designed to numb the sensation. Why? Because this will not address the underlying cause of the problem . . . and more damage may ensue. Sensitivity pastes can dull the pain felt in your teeth, especially when this involves any root dentin that may have become exposed in your mouth. These pastes frequently desensitize the tooth by creating a plug made up from a tin compound that works as a barrier substance over the exposed dentin. This will provide immediate relief, but since the underlying problem has not been addressed, more damage can occur and result in more problems elsewhere in the mouth. This is good news for the makers of solution-based toothpastes—but if you are concerned about your future oral health, these pastes are *not* your friend. The other problem with desensitizing pastes is that they may create a deposit or barrier that prevents natural healing—perhaps even *permanently*.

This is why sensitivity is better addressed by using xylitol at the end of meals, followed by a period of mouth resting (which will be explained in detail in Chapter 9). This is really a time, after using xylitol, when you do not eat or drink anything for an hour or two. This strategy allows your own saliva to heal the defects in your enamel in a natural and permanent way—not as a plug on the outside, but by helping to grow the enamel crystals and making them a more perfect shape. This is a slower process, and it may take a week or more for the sensitivity to go away—but it will be a natural repair, not fake plugging of your porous dentin or enamel. The use of my Complete Mouth Care System™ (described in Chapter Six) will help to speed up this entire process.

SPECIAL CARE SCENARIOS

Adults who experience a lack of saliva flow in their mouths are normally aware of an uncomfortable feeling of dryness. This condition, known as *dry mouth*, can be the result of many things, including: a side effect from medication; a response to prolonged stress or hormonal changes; any form of sustained physical damage from chemotherapy and/or radiation treatments; or perhaps even as the result of an autoimmune disease like Sjogren's syndrome or scleroderma, each of which can lead to circumstances where the salivary glands become dysfunctional and can no longer produce saliva.

Even those with low or absent normal production of saliva can be helped by xylitol, and it is highly recommended for people with any of these conditions—and with dosage recommendations that are the same as for *all* adults. Studies show that when xylitol is used as suggested, even for people with dry mouth, it can reduce their risk for tooth decay (in that vulnerable portion of the mouth where the root of the tooth meets the crown of the tooth) by a remarkable forty percent (40%). Patients report significant improvements in their sensation of mouth dryness when they start using xylitol, and particularly if they learn to follow it with periods of mouth resting—in place of the intermittent water sipping that we first discussed in Part One.

During the first four (4) weeks of xylitol use, you will likely notice a cleaner surface on your teeth when you look in the mirror—the result of an initial reduction in plaque. Over the next five (5) months, there will be even *less* plaque-forming bacteria in your saliva. After a solid six (6) months of xylitol use, there is normally a consistent ninety-eight percent (98%) reduction in any kind of plaque in the mouth—either on teeth or floating around in your saliva. And this can certainly be something to smile about.

MOUTH ACIDITY

Any of us can encounter the complications that accompany the presence of acid in our mouths. However, most women in particular have no idea that their dental problems can begin when they are in their teenage years, provoked by the unrecognized damage caused by mouth acidity. Hormonal shifts can cause a young female mouth to be far more acidic, and for much longer durations, than occur in healthy young male mouths. During pregnancy, women frequently encounter a variety of problems created by acidic saliva, which puts their teeth at risk for cavities and their gums at risk for gingivitis. Mouth acidity and dry mouth are the two main reasons underlying dental disease, and these problems cannot be solved by brushing, flossing, or with dental cleanings.

In addition, many people are shocked to discover how sugar-free and so-called "diet" products can contribute to cavities and promote harmful mouth bacteria, chiefly because of their acidity. Trust me when I tell you to *never* believe that a sugar-free product is *ever* safe for teeth. Diet soda, for example, can cause as much—and likely more—dental damage than a sugar-containing drink, and that is because of soda's extreme acidity. Even children's sugarless chewy vitamins or melatonin tablets can contain a dentally harmful, non-digestible substance called an *oligosaccharide*, which is classi-fied as sugar-free because it has no calories. The reason for concern around oligosaccharides is because they give energy to harmful plaque bacteria—and, in this way, they can potentially cause cavities.

Even carbonated *water* is problematic, whether sweetened or not. Adding a citrus flavor to this water will make it even more caustic to teeth, especially if it is sipped for over an hour, rather than being con-sumed within five (5) to ten (10) minutes. To protect your teeth from this kind of beverage damage known as *erosive tooth wear* (ETW), xylitol can provide a simple and effective answer. The protection is achieved as xylitol stimulates a flow of saliva that will be more alkaline than even your resting saliva. This improved or raised pH combats this acidity and neutralizes it, while also providing minerals that can help to heal any damage caused by the acidic attack.

Many people assume that baking soda is a useful product to raise one's mouth pH level, but a pH higher than 7.4 is not helpful. Baking soda creates a dissolved pH of 9—but it is baking soda's own caustic nature that strips the mouth's natural protection from tooth surfaces, leaving teeth more vulnerable to erosion, and the skin of the mouth to ulceration, and the gums to recession.

A 1970s study showed that a paste of baking soda and peroxide could eliminate an aggressive gum disease called *Acute Necrotizing Ulcerative Gingivitis* (ANUG), but the study came with a warning that prolonged use would cause gum recession and tooth sensitivity. Indeed, baking soda may clean debris off a tooth surface and make teeth immediately look whiter—but the long-term consequences of recession and tooth sensitivity should be balanced against this benefit.

To remove tooth stains, a safer method is to add a half-teaspoon ($\frac{1}{2}$ tsp.) of xylitol crystals, sprinkled over the toothpaste on your toothbrush. Target any tooth surfaces that are stained with this paste for a few days, either used alone, or as a normal part of my Complete Mouth Care System™. (See previous Chapter Six for more details on my system.) These xylitol crystals will act as an exfoliating scrub, but they will never raise the mouth pH level above 7.4.

BACTERIAL COLONIZATION IN THE MOUTH

The tension between good and bad bacteria in the mouth is clearly seen when we examine *colonization*, which is a formal term for a process whereby teeth become infected and covered by bacteria as they enter and grow as a new tooth in the mouth of a child or teenager. Hundreds of kinds of healthy bacteria generally mix with plaque bacteria and form a diverse bacterial collection, which floats throughout our mouth and is carried around in the liquid we call spit or saliva. (See Chapter Three in Part One for a fuller previous discussion of saliva.)

These floating—or *planktonic*—bacteria comprise around twenty percent (20%) of the mouth's total bacterial population, but this selection of bacteria is easily sampled with a spit test, and it can provide a good representation of the mouth's overall bacterial mix. Plaque bacteria are invisible as they float in saliva, but they become a dental problem if they multiply into visible colonies—something that can only occur if these bacteria become firmly planted on the hard, non-shedding surfaces of teeth.

Infant teeth form in the jaw before birth, but they begin to appear in the mouth around six (6) months *after* birth. The baby's saliva will flow over these teeth—and, consequently, any floating plaque-forming bacteria in this saliva will immediately land on these teeth and *colonize* the tooth surfaces. Plaque-forming bacteria latch tightly and multiply rapidly, which puts teeth at risk for developing cavities. To prevent plaque colonization from happening, it is important to clean new baby teeth as soon as you notice them in your child's mouth.

Clean Baby Teeth with Xylitol

Use a total of a quarter of a teaspoon (¼ tsp.) of xylitol each day to discourage plaque-forming bacteria from latching onto, and multiplying upon, new baby tooth surfaces. You can dissolve the xylitol crystals in an ounce of warm water and use this solution three (3) or four (4) times during the day—possibly starting after the first feeding, or at another time when your baby is awake and happy. Apply the xylitol solution with a baby toothbrush, a soft cloth, a clean glove, or something called a "finger toothbrush," which is designed to fit directly on an adult's finger so that a baby's teeth can be brushed softly and safely.

When you take this action on behalf of your baby, always make sure to reach the areas where teeth meet the gums—particularly since plaque can easily stick to the front surfaces of baby teeth, underneath the upper lip. The process should take no more than two (2) seconds and should be repeated three (3) or four (4) times daily. This will help protect baby teeth from cavities during the first years of life—something that is especially important if you are nursing your baby at night.

While xylitol works to defend baby teeth from plaque, it is also helping to nurture healthy bacteria and encourage their colonization on teeth. This becomes highly valuable, as baby molars grow and begin to break through the gum during the second year of life. New adult molar teeth will also become quickly colonized by the first bacteria to reach them, as they typically enter the child's mouth during kindergarten years. The first bacteria to enter the surface grooves of baby or adult molars will gain an advantageous foothold—and this will create a pronounced effect on the child's future oral health. This is why the earlier in time that infants and toddlers' teeth are exposed to xylitol, the better the chance that their new teeth will be colonized by healthy bacteria—and this, luckily, will only increase the child's opportunity of enjoying future oral health.

Anyone who caretakes infants or young children may also consider "cleaning" their own mouths with xylitol, in a concerted effort to decrease any chance of passing plaque-forming bacteria in saliva droplets from their mouth to those of these children. Adults should not be terrified of this risk or avoid interacting with a baby as a result. Instead, parents, family members, and caretakers should *all* actively consider steps to raise their potential for sharing healthy bacteria with their children—and capitalize on this entirely natural process of bacterial transfer, which will increase the diversity of oral bacteria in an infant's or toddler's developing mouth.

CAVITIES FOR CHILDREN AND TEENS

A consistent daily regimen of xylitol during early childhood has been shown to virtually eliminate the risk that cavities will occur in children's teeth. This has been reported in many studies but has been practically applied for over sixty years in the public health programs of European countries such as Scandinavia and Finland. Dentists have observed—and microbiological testing confirms—that if a child's mouth has cavities (caused by harmful plaque bacteria) by the age of four, this child will most likely have poor oral health as an adult. This explains the pivotal importance of baby teeth in the fight to help a child avoid cavities *early* in life.

A largely unknown (and often misinterpreted) fact is that harmful cavity bacteria travel in droplets of saliva from person to person. This is how parents with plaque, cavities, or fillings can unintentionally infect their baby's new teeth—and therefore greatly increase the likelihood of early tooth decay. The movement of harmful mouth bacteria occurs within an invisible cloud of microscopic particles that *sprays* out of our mouths whenever we talk, sing, or kiss our friends, family, or children. Teeth can never remain entirely sterile, so the goal is to nurture healthy protective bacteria that will colonize and cover baby teeth as early as possible in life.

Parents, grandparents, siblings, babysitters, and even caretakers with healthy mouths can—and *should*—share their healthy bacteria with infants and young children alike. If you are not sure about the relative state of your mouth health, there is no sense in trying to *avoid* singing a song or kissing your baby. Instead, you need only appreciate how quickly, and *easily*, plaque-forming bacteria in your mouth can be eliminated—and healthy bacteria nurtured—through the regular use of xylitol.

Ideally, a xylitol program should begin at least a few months before a baby begins to socialize widely with your family. This early preventive approach appears to control bacterial transmission and can lower a child's immediate and future risk of decay (offering protection to children even up to the ages of six to ten years old) by more than eighty (80%) percent.

This is why developing a xylitol routine is so great—even *before* pregnancy. If you want to know if xylitol is safe when you are pregnant, a study presented in 2022 clearly demonstrated its potential benefits. In that study conducted between May 2015 and October 2021—led by a team of gynecologists from Baylor University in Texas—two single-gram pieces of xylitol gum were given every day to more than 10,000 pregnant women in the East African country of Malawi, starting either before or within the first twenty (20) weeks of their pregnancy. (Pre-term birth is the leading cause of death worldwide for children under five years of age.) The women ate one piece of xylitol gum after lunch, and the second piece before going to sleep each day. While the long-term oral health of the babies was *not* a component of this study, the researchers did find a twenty-five percent (25%) decrease in the number of babies born *prematurely*—a major health challenge for the Malawi population. The pregnant women *also* noticed improvements in their *own* collective oral health—a result that the lead author of the study, Dr. Kjersti Agaard, has maintained provides the closest thing to proof that a mother's healthy mouth is linked to a lower risk of premature birth.

Another way to control plaque (as described previously in this chapter) is to brush or wipe a few xylitol crystals directly (or dissolved in water) onto baby teeth, starting as soon as they emerge into the mouth. If you have missed the chance to introduce xylitol into your family early in your child's life, don't worry—there are more opportunities to do so.

For example, a good time is as a child begins to eat solid foods at the age of two (2)—the start of what is known as the *toddler stage.* Soft xylitol mints in child-appropriate flavors can be eaten at the end of meals, and again before sleep time. It is safe and beneficial to have these mints *after* brushing teeth, as this will ensure that your child's mouth is protected during the night—especially if tooth brushing becomes a struggle. Studies show that the regular use of xylitol may also help to reduce the risk of otitis media ear infections for a child, which is an especially painful problem that can often occur during this stage of childhood.

The next window of opportunity to impact your child's oral health is at the *kindergarten stage,* around the age of five (5) or six (6), when new adult molar teeth begin to grow—or erupt—into the mouth. Both baby and adult molar teeth have a wide and crinkled biting surface. The grooves and pits in these teeth are home to critical bacteria, so it is crucial to ensure that these are *healthy* bacteria and not cavity-forming ones. This is why it is prudent to introduce xylitol into your child's daily routine prior to the appearance of these molars—ideally, six (6) months *before* they enter the mouth. When deep grooves of molars are populated by healthy bacteria, this preferred state can help protect future adult teeth and help promote a more permanently stable bacterial population in your child's mouth.

When children use xylitol *early* in life and consider oral care as enjoyable and fun, this can be a wonderful foundation for future dental experiences. The final adult teeth—the *wisdom* teeth—often find their way into the mouth later in *adolescence* and *teendom* (9–19 years old), and sometimes even later. This is a time when plaque transmission can be a problem, shared between teens who have less than perfect oral care habits. Wisdom teeth are hard to access, and they grow slowly and often at a strange angle, making them difficult to clean.

This can also be a time when your teen may have less interest in caring for his or her teeth. Gum disease can begin around any adult tooth, and certain periodontal bacteria secrete a substance that dissolves in water to make it taste foul. Stop your teen from spiraling down the road to periodontal disease if they dislike the taste of water, and before they become hooked on stronger tasting and more mouth-damaging energy or soda drinks, which can make cavity and gum problems worse—and potentially cause exaggerated issues that may involve their digestive health or impact sinus, ear, and/or respiratory health.

Teens usually love the delicious flavors of xylitol gum and mints, which will always be useful—although for ideal mouth health, it is better (as discussed in Chapter Six) to combine xylitol with my Complete Mouth Care System™. What matters most, of course, is that they are guided in the right way so that they come to regard oral health care as a necessary—and even *enjoyable*—part of their life.

REVERSAL OF CAVITIES

Long-term studies undertaken in the Belize region of Central America from 1989 to 1994 were able to document how cavities in some of the study subjects had reversed during the study period. Careful examination indicated that tooth decay stabilized in the xylitol group—in both the outer tooth enamel and inner dentin—and, in some of the cases, the cavities had completely healed.

Arguments from dental authorities in the United States claimed these studies lacked a control group. This would have been a group of children given sugar to eat, so as to show the differences between their teeth and the xylitol group. Obviously, this was not a possibility, but many years ago the University of Turku (mentioned earlier in Chapter Seven) navigated the problem and created equipment called a *caries model*—an artificial mouth with real teeth and saliva. Sugar was introduced and cavities formed, as opposed to the other mouth that was contrasted with the results obtained if xylitol was used to prevent cavities.

All of this should prove one thing to you—just because your dentist hasn't offered you a home-based solution to your tooth and gum issues doesn't mean that there isn't one. There *is*, and I hope that now you feel confident to explore xylitol in your own family.

CONCLUSION

Life and unexpected career choices have exposed me to an interesting series of varied dental experiences. My compassion for phobic patients, and the fortunate discovery of a solution to dental problems, has directed me to teach this strategy for decades. My Complete Mouth Care System™ allows people to experience a change in their mouth health and a way to sustain this improvement day after day.

In the next chapter, we are going to explore what I like to call the Four Keys to Preventive Mouth Care. To get an even firmer grasp on what's happening around and between the molars, canines, and incisors that make up your smile, read on!

9

$\mathscr{T}$he Four Keys to
Preventive Mouth Care—
Unlocking All the Doors

The eye is the window of the soul, the mouth the door.
—HIRAM POWERS, NINETEENTH-CENTURY AMERICAN SCULPTOR

I magine that you find yourself in a barren corridor with nothing but four doors—all locked against you. Desperate to break free from this confinement, you reach into your pocket and discover a set of four invaluable keys that can unlock *all* the doors . . . and provide you with unencumbered access to the wonderful castle beyond that hallway. Now consider the castle as a healthy mouth; the hallway as the isolated trap of dental disease; and those four keys as the priceless steps toward better oral care that I am now about to share with you.

The following four keys are valuable ideas that can improve your dental health for the rest of your life. Does this sound like an exciting opportunity you are eager to take, or does it scare you to consider that you may need to make changes? If you are feeling unsure about trying something new for your dental issues, don't beat yourself up over this. After all, new concepts often bring uncertainty, but that is why you have already been presented in earlier chapters with descriptions of the way teeth repair; the usefulness of good mouth bacteria; and all the *whys* and *wherefores* concerning cavities and gum disease.

These four keys that follow are solutions to give you a way out from ongoing dental treatments, and a pathway so that you can become empowered to control the environment in your mouth—and achieve the outcome you desire for your oral health.

WHAT *ARE* THE FOUR KEYS?

These keys are concepts that will assist you to stop, prevent, and even reverse problematic disease in your mouth so you will have a life with no more painful cavities or destructive gum disease—problems that have affected people around the world since the dawn of civilization. You *can* prevent cavities before they start, and you do not need to allow fillings to fail, drilling to *kill* your teeth, or gum disease to *fester* in your mouth. And it is entirely rational for you to be wary of the way our current dental paradigm allows older citizens to experience increasing dental expenses and worsening oral health as they age—issues that may contribute to chronic inflammatory health problems and impact their overall enjoyment of life.

Each key is one of four critical components that impact oral health. Some of this advice may be in opposition to instructions you have been given by your dentist or hygienist, and I know many people who love their dentist too much to contradict them, question them, or take a different approach on their own. If this is your situation, perhaps read this chapter and simply *take notes*. You can then bring your findings with you to discuss at your next dental visit.

My goal is to help you develop a strategy for dental health—making simple changes that boost your success and that make the journey more enjoyable. You will quickly notice how these puzzle pieces intertwine and connect. I will not repeat information about my Complete Mouth Care System™ or xylitol, since these have been described respectively in Chapters Six and Seven. Instead, we will look at how to achieve oral health in a more universal and—for those who live *outside* the US—globally accessible format. This chapter will be useful for people in countries where the products named in my system are not necessarily available. The hope is that this advice will be useful for *everyone* who wants improved mouth health.

This is why we are going to address:

- How to clean your teeth (*effective daily oral care*);

- The power of saliva to improve oral health (*mouth resting*);

- What to eat (*healthy diet and meals*); and

- Body healing (*digestion, immune health, and stem cell science*)

THE FOUR KEYS

The following offers concepts and protocols that touch on areas of science in general—and biochemistry, in particular—that will likely go beyond what you may or may *not* already know. It is important, however, to have an idea of these core concepts as they are part of the reason *why* my strategy of mouth care works so effectively. After all, what goes on in your mouth will be served even better by what you understand and believe in your head—and I feel privileged to share some of this interesting science with you here in this book.

So, here we go!

KEY 1—EFFECTIVE DAILY ORAL CARE

The products you choose for your oral care need not only to address harmful plaque on the surfaces of your teeth—they should also target plaque *formation* and the immature plaque bacteria that float in saliva. If you can stop the sticky buildup that causes damage to teeth and gums, that's always a good thing. But it is really important that we preserve and develop a population of healthy mouth bacteria during this process—which involves a delicate balance that is not always easy to achieve.

The world of oral care is controlled mainly by large companies that design toothpaste and other products to work like medications for your teeth—formulated and sold to you as a one-stop-shop to deal with the *symptoms* of dental disease, while doing nothing to combat the underlying *cause*. For years now, people in America have seen innumerable advertisements and toothpaste packaging with language that suggests every different paste on the market is the *only* one needed to end mouth sensitivity, whiten teeth, or help fight against existing periodontal or gum disease. There are no products out there that suggest they will help *prevent* problems—just products to reduce the pain and keep you happy . . . for a time.

A well-designed toothpaste and/or mouthrinse should accelerate the absorption of minerals into your teeth, no matter if you have sensitivity, cavities, discolored teeth, or gum disease. You don't want a putty-style filler to block up open pores in your teeth or a whitening paste that removes minerals and can change the protein structure of your tooth. As I suggested in Chapter Six, try to look for a simple toothpaste made with silica—and, ideally, one that contains sodium fluoride listed on the product label at a low concentration of 0.24%. (This kind of weight percentage is normally reported on the label to describe how much sodium fluoride there would be in a hundred grams of this kind of toothpaste.)

Try to avoid glycerin, if possible, since this may interfere with mineralization and reversal of cavities. A good mouth rinse should *also* not contain glycerin, and I recommend a rinse with a dilute concentration of sodium fluoride around 0.05% (which, like the toothpaste, indicates an amount of sodium fluoride in the liquid). Keep in mind that sodium fluoride is a relatively expensive ingredient, so you must pay attention and look for its presence in oral care products—and, of course, *always* avoid stannous fluoride, a much less expensive tin-based compound that I *do not* recommend.

An excellent toothbrush will do more for bleeding gums, and to help heal gum pockets, than any aggressive toothpaste you may find marketed for gum disease. Look for a toothbrush with plenty of resilient bristles of different lengths (often called a *flossing brush*). This kind of brush will make a difference, especially if you use a proper and consistent technique of gum massage following the directions that I presented in Chapter Six. A top-quality toothbrush will help to stimulate circulation in your gums and initiate the healing response that will make the difference between periodontal success and failure.

I also advise that you reconsider any expensive electric brush that you *think* is helping you—it is highly likely that it *isn't*. Test one or two good manual brushes and see if they feel better for your gums. You may be surprised to discover that a well-designed manual brush is far superior to the more expensive sonic varieties.

KEY 2—MOUTH RESTING

In general, the biggest problem for teeth is our culture's incessant habit of sipping beverages—and snacking between meals. The trouble at play here is the elimination of the time when saliva would normally repair teeth from the damage that acidity causes whenever we eat and/or drink. Generally, you will want to give your mouth a rest for at least an hour after every meal—avoiding the sipping of *anything*, even water—so that your mouth can recover and restore a healthy balance. The quality of our saliva matters, and there are several ways to improve it.

Exercise and Mouth Health

Any body movement—whether it is yoga, walking, pickleball, dancing, running, or rowing—will help generate improved saliva production in the mouth. When we are happy and relaxed, it appears that a tranquil state of mind *also* benefits the quality of saliva to some degree, and there is also an impact from things we eat, read, watch, consider, and do—even an impact from our social circles and experiences of love. Our saliva dries up or flows more under the direction of many influences, and many studies have shown that simply being *grateful* for food can alter the composition and flow rate of saliva as we *look* at food.

Studies from both Kings College in London, England and the University of Miami in Florida—conducted between the years 2017 and 2020—have shown some interesting things about saliva. For example, it was discovered that the more rapidly our saliva flows, the better we will sense the aroma of the food—and the more ability we each will have to enjoy its taste.

Stress and anger can create a variety of negative health outcomes, and these emotions can also decrease salivary flow and increase tooth damage. A dry mouth environment—especially one that is acidic— will promote more damage and disease. In Part One, we discussed the value of the saliva (or "spit") in our mouth—in particular, we established that the longer we can allow it to interact with our mouth after meals, the better it is for mouth health. And based on what we examined in Chapter Seven, saliva that is stimulated by even one or two grams of *xylitol* will lead to a far healthier mouth bacteria—so I advise you to again consider xylitol as a great benefit at the end of meals, and before periods of mouth resting.

The Salivary Circle of Mouth Health

Many people feel challenged to resist eating and drinking for an hour after meals, especially when they first adopt this habit. In light of this struggle, I need to explain why I will next suggest that—for ideal health—we *double* this period of mouth resting. To understand why, we will explore a specific interaction that occurs between certain mouth bacteria, healthy saliva, and nutrients absorbed by the body when we eat green leafy vegetables. This chain of events is something I call the *salivary circle of mouth health*.

This interaction will not occur well unless the mouth is populated by healthy oral bacteria, and only if saliva carries these special nutrients—called *nitrates*—that are absorbed from foods. (These nitrates will be absorbed best when you have a healthy gut, and only when we consume specific foods such as fruits, like strawberries, and vegetables, including celery, lettuce, red and green spinach, and beets.)

When nitrates leave the gut, they are then carried by the blood circulation to the salivary glands and into saliva—a coordinated event that requires management by a healthy immune system. When you have a healthy body, this complex circle of events occurs smoothly, and this allows the saliva in the mouth to become a valuable resource for our gums and teeth. For those who employ mouth resting a little longer, one additional reaction can turn these nitrates into an almost *magical* compound for our body health—extending saliva's healing benefits to help our breathing, heart, and brain health. Let me next explain how this happens, and why you can only derive these benefits when you provide saliva with sixty (60) to ninety (90) minutes of mouth resting, after meals.

Denitrifying Bacteria

A large international study called the Human Microbiome Project of 2007 (which we already first discussed in Chapter One) showed surprising things about human bodies that shocked many doctors and dentists. The results illustrated an enormous variety of previously unrecognized bacteria on and inside the human body and revealed that a healthy mouth can house over eight hundred (800) different kinds of oral bacteria. An elite group of these bacteria appear to form a central community on our tongue surface, and they support and appear to organize other healthy bacteria. The total population of bacteria in our mouth will vary in type from tooth to tooth, and from location to location, with specific kinds found in niche areas—but together, if they create a diverse and well-functioning microbiological ecology, this is called a healthy oral *microbiome.*

When you have a healthy oral microbiome, the bacteria on your tongue will have a special ability to interact with those compounds in your saliva called *nitrates.* An hour or so after we have eaten nitrate-containing foods, these bacteria on our tongue interact with nitrates in saliva and turn them into new compounds called *nitrites.* This community of bacteria on our tongue are not only important for mouth health but for changing nitrates into nitrites. And *this* is why they are known collectively as *denitrifying bacteria*—because the term describes specifically their ability to denitrify any nitrates in saliva.

The next stage of this process occurs when we swallow these nitrites that form on the tongue. When these compounds reach our stomach, they react with our stomach acids to form a gas called *nitric oxide*. The *key* reason that this interaction is important is because nitric oxide has a direct effect on our lungs, heart, and brain health. It is absorbed into the nearby body areas, causing the walls of important breathing tubes and blood vessels to relax—a reaction that allows more blood to flow through them. Within seconds of this absorption, nitric oxide directly benefits our breathing and goes on to improve our heart and brain health. Studies show that nitric oxide also has a powerful and beneficial effect on our nervous system, our daily sleep-wake cycle, and our hormone health.

Nitric oxide gas is also produced in the nose, where it is stored in the small and large sinus caverns that wind throughout the bones in the front and middle of our face. Healthy sinuses release nitric oxide every time we breathe through our nose, while chronically infected sinuses can instead cause a *depletion* of nitric oxide. This, of course, leads to an overall imbalance in the body—and, once again, this is why I recommend the use of a xylitol-based nasal spray, which will help keep your nasal passages as healthy and *clear* as possible.

To check your own nitric oxide levels, you can use nitric oxide test strips. When you coat these paper sticks with saliva, a color is generated that you can match with a related chart intended to help *indicate* the nitric oxide levels in your mouth. Be aware, however, that these levels should be measured at least an hour or two *after* eating. If you cannot generate a very pale color on the test strip, which indicates a low level of nitric oxide, consider how nitric oxide production is affected by poor mouth or digestive health, diet, and/or by chronic sinus problems. Nitric oxide will *also* be reduced if you happen to take any medications that may dry out your mouth, such as allergy and/or blood pressure medications.

Nitric oxide production is also affected by chemotherapy and radiation treatment, and it is prevented by acid reflux medications (like, for example, proton pump inhibitors) since too little stomach acid will shut down nitric oxide production. Talk with your doctor about foods that can jumpstart stomach health; foods rich in zinc and vitamin B_{12} (red meat, fish, soy, dairy, seeds, and whole grains), and also in iodine (seafood, tuna, eggs, and the already-mentioned dairy). Fermented foods like sauerkraut and pickles can also be useful.

Something to Think About

This is a good moment to point out that there are *still* some "myths" on the Internet that *suggest* how nitric oxide production is reduced by using mouthwash because it reduces denitrifying bacteria on the tongue. This assertion is, as you might already have guessed, incorrect and does not apply to the oral care products and strategies that I recommend.

Harnessing the power of saliva for mouth health is a new concept for many, but we should now be able to see how nutrients in foods work to protect vital body functions through an extraordinary oral pathway. We can begin to appreciate the importance of our dietary choices, and how crucial it is to give our mouth an adequate amount of resting time after meals. Hopefully, the remarkable salivary circle of health that I have described for you here can help you to enjoy nutritious meals that offer many health benefits, including a boost for our breathing, circulation, and cognitive function.

KEY 3—HEALTHY DIET (AND MEALS)

Most people know sugar is bad for teeth, but few people understand *how* it negatively impacts teeth. Sugar does its primary damage by feeding any plaque bacteria into our mouth, and it supplies them with energy to damage our oral health. Many people try to eliminate sugar from their diet to prevent cavities, and this is rarely a pathway to success.

The problem is that if plaque bacteria exist in the mouth, then decay and gum disease will always be possible consequences. In addition, many foods that we do not think of as sweet contain *hidden* sugars. Lowering our intake of sugary foods may be a good overall strategy for health, but *completely* excluding "sugars" from your diet is close to impossible—and this total restriction is *not* my recommendation, either for health or as a practical way to change your oral health.

Carbohydrates, for example, are instantly digested and broken down to form sugars in the mouth—even *before* they are swallowed. This makes all carbohydrates—from potatoes to bread—possible sources of sugar, hidden or not. More surprising sources of carbohydrate or sugars will include an array of vegetables; additives in vitamins (substances known as *oligosaccharides*); and a confusing list of sweeteners, even some that are billed as "zero calorie" but that still support plaque acid production. This particular list of occurring sugars encompasses most everyday condiments, like mustard and ketchup; many commercially available varieties of canned and fresh fruit products; most processed and prepackaged foods (even those created for kids and babies); yogurts; and, of course, the typical assemblage of chocolates, chewing gums, crackers, baked goods, and cookies that most of us would assume is a direct source of danger for your teeth and gums.

What makes this sugar equation such a consistent and *uphill* battle is that you only need a few grains of sugar to jumpstart the harmful activity of plaque in your mouth—or, said another way, the *quantity* of sugar you consume is not as important for mouth health as the *frequency* and *duration* of time during which sugar is in your mouth. This is why a more successful approach is to plan healthy meals, and then *end* every meal with a tooth-protective food or—you guessed it—xylitol, which will negate any drop in your mouth's pH level generated by the sugary foods and/or beverages in question.

This said, certain foods can certainly be classified as the *worst* for teeth, and they are any foods that have a texture that causes them to stick onto—or *into*—the crevices of teeth. Many crackers and breakfast cereals can stick around or on teeth, and these are often treats that we give to the young children in our lives.

Remember that most of these crackers do not *seem* sweet or look, at first glance, like a tooth-decaying danger. Carbohydrates, as mentioned, quickly turn into sugar in the mouth—and if a piece of food attaches itself to a tooth or is squeezed into the grooves of teeth, this gives harmful plaque bacteria a long duration to feed . . . and create damaging acids all the while. This is why sticky or highly processed foods, especially soft cereals and crackers, are particularly dangerous for teeth. If you and/or your children tend to snack on cookies, cereal, or crackers—especially late in the evening, when your saliva flow is reduced—you need to be aware that this habit can *ruin teeth*.

The speed at which you will notice positive change in your mouth will depend on how well you keep to this routine of meal "times," which will drastically limit how much damage your mouth experiences each day. Other factors—such as smoking cigarettes; having a dry mouth, either from allergy medications or as a side effect from prescribed drugs; treatments for hormone deficiency; chronic sinus infections; or continual stress—can work against you and slow your progress. Our mouth chemistry ultimately ends up being as unique and individual as we are in life—but there *are* certain foods that can help us overcome these unwanted effects . . . and *also* help our saliva become more beneficial to fight this fight.

The following are foods that should be included in an ideal diet to: improve saliva quality; augment and support our immune system; and positively impact the speed of tooth and gum repair, even as it promotes overall healing within your body.

Water-rich Foods

Carrots, celery, cucumber, apples, and melons are all water-rich and fibrous foods that help to keep the mouth hydrated while they also boost saliva production. Tomatoes and pink grapefruit contain special nutrients called *bioactives*, which can protect the DNA of cells from damage that may occur during X-rays, provided that they are consumed *prior* to any radiation. Medical imaging of any kind can deliver radiation with the potential to traumatize the DNA of healthy cells in the body—and also to cause a malfunction if these genes are repeatedly damaged.

Key Foods for the Health of Your Teeth and Mouth

Water-rich Foods

These foods all help to keep the mouth hydrated, boost saliva production, and contain high levels of special nutrients called *bioactives* that are able to protect the DNA of cells from any damage that may occur during X-rays (provided that they are consumed *prior* to any radiation).

Apples	Cucumbers	Pink Grapefruit
Carrots	Melons	Tomatoes
Celery		

Calcium-rich Foods

These foods are good for bone and tooth health, and contain many nutrients (including vitamins A and B_{12}, potassium, magnesium, and iodine) that can *also* help improve saliva health.

Cheese	Whole Milk
Kefir *(see Yogurts)*	Yogurts *(see Kefir)*

Foods Rich in Vitamins and Antioxidants

All these delicious natural foods contain various levels of the vitamins A, B_6, C, and E, together with health-promoting *beta-carotene* and *magnesium*. Working as powerful antioxidants, they help to boost immune and mouth health in a variety of ways.

Bananas	Pineapple
Blueberries	Raspberries

Fresh apples are a great example of a food rich in probiotic properties (together with the aforementioned bioactives) that help to speed up the repair of DNA damage to reduce damaging effects. This is why apples are useful when they are consumed *after* one has undergone X-rays, or for patients with disrupted salivary glands

Leafy salad vegetables (and greens)	Seeds
Nuts	Strawberries
Papaya	Sweet Potatoes

Foods for Dry Mouth and/or Bad Breath

Garlic and onions contain a naturally occurring compound called *allicin* that aids in saliva production, nourishes our immune system, and supports the bacteria that help to ward off bad breath. Both ginger and mushrooms can help with dry mouth and remain a great source of immunity-stimulating dietary fiber along with *bioactives* (mentioned above) for an overall improvement of digestive health.

Garlic	Mushrooms
Ginger	Onions

Anti-inflammatory, Anti-viral, and Anti-bacterial

Turmeric (which contains curcumin) and green tea can help to lower and control body inflammation by virtue of certain plant compounds they contain that are called *flavonoids*. These flavonoids provide a number of beneficial health effects that protect our body and reduce our risk for disease. Meanwhile, many types of shellfish can boost our immune health, and oyster, crab, and lobster are especially high in zinc—an element that supports our immune function, which helps the body fight viruses and bacteria.

Crab	Oyster
Curcumin *(see Turmeric)*	Shellfish
Green tea	Turmeric *(see Curcumin)*
Lobster	

who are following a course of radiation and/or chemotherapy. Apples can *also* help anyone who develops a sore tongue and/or mouth after long dental treatments—and I will sometimes suggest that these patients first shred an apple into fine slivers with a kitchen grater, to make it softer and easier to consume.

Calcium-rich Foods

Cheese and whole milk are rich in calcium and phosphorus, minerals that are *both* good for bone and tooth health. Dairy-rich foods also contain many nutrients (including vitamin A, B$_{12}$, potassium, magnesium and iodine) that can *also* help improve saliva health and help to heal teeth. High-quality yogurts (including a variety of yogurt referred to as *kefir*, usually consumed as a drink because its consistency is thinner than that of more conventional yogurt products) are *also* rich in calcium alongside their probiotic properties—and this helps not only to improve a body's digestive and immune health, but also aids in balancing oral health and production of saliva.

Foods for Dry Mouth and/or Bad Breath

Onions (along with its close cousin, garlic) contain a naturally occurring chemical compound called *allicin*, which boosts saliva production and benefits immune health—and goes on to have a positive impact on gum health. Consider the following: Researchers at the University of Florida have conducted a variety of studies looking at the benefits of foods on health—and in 2016, they showed the effect of aged garlic on the immune system of healthy men and women during the cold and flu season. Blood analysis showed a supercharged response in the immune cells of those who ate the garlic.

In addition, the natural spice ginger stimulates saliva production directly and can be helpful for people with a dry mouth while it also supports the immune system. Mushrooms, meanwhile, are a great source of immunity-stimulating dietary fiber along with certain nutrients called bioactives (mentioned earlier) for an overall improvement of digestive health.

Vitamins and Antioxidants for Healthy Biofilm

Leafy salad vegetables and greens are rich in vitamins A, C, and E, all of which are powerful antioxidants that help to boost immune health.

(They also provide nitrates that improve saliva quality.) Nuts and seeds offer a source of valuable nutrients for oral health, including proteins, antioxidants, magnesium for salivary health, and vitamin E. Sweet potatoes are especially high in the pigment-producing element known as *beta-carotene*, which can be converted into vitamin A that has been shown to support skin and mouth health. Bananas are rich in magnesium and vitamin B$_6$, which can help improve sleep, while this popular fruit's fiber *also* supports immune health. Papaya and pineapple are two unique fruits for digestive health, each contributing enzymes that can be a help to those who experience acid reflux. Small amounts of these fruits can be eaten right before a meal as an appetizer—which allows these enzymes to help support improved upper digestive health.

Why is this important? Because the process helps to reduce the unpleasant and painful symptoms of acid or gastric reflux—a problem that negatively influences mouth health in many ways, especially as it can cause erosion of teeth and promotion of unhealthy mouth conditions. Berries of all kinds—blueberries, strawberries, and raspberries among others—are rich in antioxidants and vitamin C, and they all contain some naturally occurring xylitol. Studies have shown that berries have a particularly useful impact on mouth health and help to develop protective biofilm over teeth.

Anti-inflammatory, Anti-viral, and Anti-bacterial

Turmeric (which contains curcumin) and green tea can help to lower and control body inflammation by virtue of certain plant compounds they contain that are called *flavonoids*. These compounds provide a number of beneficial health effects that protect our body and reduce our risk for disease. One way this occurs is through the antioxidant properties of the flavonoids, which enhance our immune system and mouth health—and, consequently, our gum health.

Shellfish can boost saliva health, while oyster, crab, and lobster are each high in zinc—and these *all* support immune function, while helping the body fight viruses and bacteria.

Food Pairing

The nutrients in foods can be better absorbed by the body through the application of a relatively new concept called *food pairing*. This involves the discovery that we can enhance our nutrition by eating certain foods *in combination* with other foods, and in patterns that extract more benefits from these foods. Generally, we will have optimal absorption when these partner foods are eaten or paired as a meal since they interact and trigger reactions that provide us with maximum absorption of the nutrients in each.

There are many examples of this kind of food pairing—for example, eating banana with some dairy product (like yogurt, milk, custard, or kefir) can allow the fiber in the banana to support the gut bacteria that digest dairy, and the outcome will be enhanced calcium uptake. This method allows us to increase the nutritional value of our diet to a level that is higher than the sum of eating each food individually—and this allows us to reap additional health benefits.

The possibilities are endless and most combinations on a dinner plate will be a balanced mixture of colors that taste good together, which should encourage us *all* to opt for meal-style eating. There are also benefits in high fiber and fermented food diets that help more minerals to be absorbed by the and it appears better if we consume sugary foods at the end of meals, to allow fibrous foods (vegetables, grains, and legumes) to be digested *first*, as the fiber-utilizing bacteria will gain energy and promote improved digestion and absorption of all the nutrients. A practical application of this kind of food paring would be to eat an apple or some kiwi fruit (each high in fiber) *before* a sugary cookie or muffin.

The types of foods—together with the order in which we consume them—remain important to our mouth health. However, the daily process of eating should never become overly complicated by science. For instance, let's consider the work of Erica and Justin Sonnenberg, senior researchers at the Stanford Center for Clinical Research in California. This married couple have studied how different diets affect our general health for more than twenty years. Erica passionately teaches how foods are a powerful lever to fight disease and improve health—and in 2021, colleagues of theirs at the Stanford Nutrition Studies Research Group published the so-called "FeFiFo" (Fermented Fiber Foods) study. Thirty-six (36) individuals ate diets with more fermented, or fiber-rich foods, added to every meal. The results showed rapid changes as their gut bacteria adapted—in some cases, within twenty (20) minutes.

Erica Sonnenberg says we can enjoy so many benefits by consistently adding some active-culture, or fermented and fiber-rich foods, to our meals—perhaps with a side of sauerkraut or colorful veggies. In service to that concept, here below are some food combinations to consider:

Tomatoes with Olive Oil

When tomatoes are consumed with olive oil, the *healthy* fat in the oil encourages the release of a compound called *lycopene* from the tomato. Its release then makes the combination of these two foods more effective at reducing unwanted chemical toxins throughout the body.

Citrus Fruits with Spinach

When vitamin C-rich foods (such as citrus fruits like lemons and/or oranges) are squeezed onto a vegetable dish like spinach, more of the iron in the spinach will more readily be absorbed.

Avocado and Carrots / Salad Greens with an Egg

When an avocado is eaten alongside carrots, more of a specific carotenoid molecule called *beta-carotene* will be absorbed from the carrots, and certain carotenoids can also convert into vitamin A. When an egg is consumed alongside carotenoid-containing salad greens, researchers at Purdue University in 2015 discovered in their study that three (3) to nine (9) times more carotenoids were absorbed into the body from the salad greens with an egg . . . as opposed to when the greens were eaten alone.

Other Food Pairings

There are many other food pairings that *also* offer health benefits, and you may wish to access any number of free online videos and webinars (some by Erica Sonnenberg or Dr. William Li, who teach about nutrition for health) or draw from any/all available Internet searches to discover food combinations that you may enjoy. Wonderful examples of culinary pairing include: Oatmeal and berries; broccoli and mustard; beans and rice; salmon and broccoli; eggs and spinach; chickpeas and lemon juice; and let's not forget the famous combination found at the Wimbledon Tennis tournament tea gardens, fresh strawberries with cream. Yum!

KEY 4. DIGESTION, IMMUNE HEALTH, AND STEM CELL SCIENCE

In this section, we will explore a new way to think about disease and wellness, and how they exist in a kind of perpetual *tension* within the body. Disease—and its associated damage—can position itself to tip our health balance, but with the help of delicious foods and a few smart lifestyle choices, we can *tilt* this scale back to our favor— toward the side of repair, regeneration, and optimal wellness. This process of balance mirrors the way teeth and gums are protected from damage and disease by preventive daily care and habits. In the same way, our body will be healthier if we limit damage and support our body's amazing self-healing system. Good daily habits make a difference, but toxins and infection will burden our body's repair machinery; the essential mechanism by which we maintain and improve body health.

New Molecular Medicine

Molecular medicine is a branch of medicine that studies how diseases, medicines, and foods either help or harm us—by looking at how they interact with different cells in our body. This approach helps to discern more clearly what is occurring inside us at a molecular level—something that has been impossible until recently. Molecular science has witnessed remarkable cell interactions and capability— some that must have been an experience as awesome as that encountered by Dutch scientist Antonie van Leeuwenhoek in 1674, when he first saw plaque (collected from his own teeth) under a microscope and noticed little animals in the lens . . . particles that were, in fact, plaque bacteria scrutinized under magnification. New discoveries can be astounding, but so is the fact that today—more than three hundred years later—most people *still* don't know that tooth plaque is a seething mass of bacteria.

Perhaps this is the first time you have heard of molecular medicine, and you may be in for some surprises. Molecular medicine has helped scientists learn how the body can rid itself of disease, and how the nutrients called *bioactives* (see earlier in this chapter) in certain foods can stimulate the body's own repair and regeneration systems. Scientists have watched the movie-like process that occurs as new blood vessels grow into transportation systems, fully equipped to deliver ready-to-help cells to areas of the body that need healing and repair . . . and this process is how your gums can repair in your mouth. You may not be excited by science, and perhaps you want to know if it is necessary to learn about mouth acidity and bacteria, or can you simply follow the directions and heal your teeth and gums. This is a good question, and the answer is yes—the results will be great—whether you know the science or not.

Wound Healing

When a body part is injured, it sends out an emergency chemical—a kind of distress signal that then triggers a wave of coordinated reactions that together are referred to by science professionals as a *healing response*. This highly coordinated pattern of events allows the body to clean up and build new tissues in a wounded area. If, however, a bodily infection *blocks* this signal or the healing response is compromised, then these events *cannot* occur as nature intends.

Stem Cells and *Angiogenesis*

Stem cells are part of an organized healing system housed within our body. Just as the development of a baby in the uterus is a coordinated dance that involves the development of body parts from stem cells, so also, from the first day we are born, stem cells travel throughout our body to repair any organs or part of our body in need. After birth, humans have a supply of about seventy (70) million or more of these cells held in reservoirs around the body, and they serve us throughout life. What we must realize is that as we age, these stem cell reservoirs can become depleted. The good news is that specific foods and lifestyles energize stem cells—and even stimulate the formation of *new* ones.

The stem cells involved in gum healing can be summoned by gum massage to contribute to a healing response that can regrow new gums, periodontal attachments (the fibers between teeth and the jawbone), and even new bone around teeth. The main thing stem cells need is a circulating fluid to carry them to the location of need. If a blood supply is missing, this is when the complex and miraculous mechanism known as *angiogenesis* kicks in.

You may have been told by your dentist that your gums or the bone around your teeth cannot heal or regrow—and this is correct information, if you have plaque or an infection in the gum pocketing around your teeth. These infections from plaque and periodontal bacteria will prevent the transmission of the signals and healing response that result in regrowth of your gums.

Here's the good news—xylitol eliminates plaque, and my Complete Mouth Care System™ will help your gum pockets heal. If you have had gum problems for some time, it is reasonable to assume that your body's warning signals are not being received—and that this infection is preventing repair. Our body tires of chronic or ongoing signaling when it is unable to properly respond, as this creates a challenging and frequently chronic health condition known as *inflammation*.

Angiogenesis is the growth of new blood capillaries from existing blood vessels. The new blood vessels are then able to carry the needed stem cells to the area that has been damaged. In the first step of angiogenesis, cells push themselves through the wall of the blood vessel that housed them, and in the process, they are flattened. Once outside the wall of the blood vessel, the cell curls into a tube shape and become the first part of a new blood capillary.

As one cell after another joins this sequence, the blood vessel grows and becomes a functional transport for the stem cells to move into an area of need. Once stem cells have reached the wounded area, they change again, but this time into the tissue that the body requires. This phenomenon can occur after a heart attack, to heal a broken bone, a skin wound and, more to the point of this book, as and when you need new gum or bone to grow around your teeth.

You may now be asking yourself, *Why is a knowledge of stem cells so important when it comes to your oral health?* The answer is that we need stem cells to heal our gums and the skin of our mouth *every day.* Natural wear and tear happens whenever we eat and drink, but any problems from these activities will be avoided if we can compensate for this damage by proactively engaging stem cells to heal our gums and regenerate them daily.

The first stage of gum healing involves the growth of new blood vessels through a process called *angiogenesis.* These new blood vessels allow transportation of special cells to regrow your gums—and these are known as *stem cells.*

Foods to Support Wound Healing

Specific foods stimulate an improved wound response, and some of these foods include: Dark chocolate (which can *stimulate* stem cells); black and green teas (which can *mobilize* stem cells); grains (especially barley); and seeds (including flax, sunflower, pumpkin, and chia), all of which can speed up the process of angiogenesis to bring a needed blood flow to the gums. Herbs like rosemary, peppermint, and ginseng can be useful, as well as the fruit and peels of fresh apples and plums, which help the repair process. Capers and onions, dried cherries, sultana raisins, and blueberries are similarly beneficial for wound healing.

The problem, of course, is that quantifying the amount of food for this beneficial effect on wound healing has not yet been completed—and in many cases, there is no absolute confirmation of their effectiveness. We have studies, however, that show a higher number of circulating stem cells in the blood of people with a lower risk for developing heart and other health problems. Conversely, a low level of stem cells in blood is linked with arthritis and chronic diseases. So, you can decide whether you want to wait for confirmation of these studies or decide—like *me*—that if eating some chocolate with a cup of tea can activate healing stem cells . . . then why *wait*?

CONCLUSION

As we have established throughout this book, the human body has its own amazing inbuilt ability to heal. Xylitol, coupled with my Complete Mouth Care System™, stand as powerful partners to boost the outcomes for your gums and teeth. If, however, the products named in my system are not available, the four key strategies described in this chapter will be good companions for you.

It is time for you to take charge of your oral health and stop any ongoing craziness of the never-ending dental fillings or treatments that you may up to now have merely accepted as your lot in life. Instead, appreciate how our bodies are amazing healing machines, and how they have the power to rid the body of the bacteria, viruses, and nasty chemicals that try to derail us. With benefit of what you have learned here in this chapter, you now have an open door—and the *keys*—that you will need to turn things around both for your mouth and your overall body health.

Even with all the knowledge that has been provided in these pages, you may *still* find yourself in a place where you and your mouth are on *one* side of the fence—and your dentist is on the *other*.

What follows in the next chapter are some steps and strategies to help you reinvent a better relationship with dentistry—and suggestions about how to maintain a healthy connection with your current or a new dentist; to enjoy future dental appointments; and to reap the benefits that these can offer.

My hope is that you will overcome fears and use this new knowledge of what is possible for you to do for yourself . . . to feel empowered, to dispel any dental angst, and create the opportunity for dental visits to become periodic evaluations that are informative and interesting. There are so many reasons for oral care to be a positive and meaningful core health value, and my hope is that we can welcome a new era of patient empowerment, drill- and injection-free dental offices, new ways to limit fear, improved patient attitudes, and a more open and enjoyable access to dentistry. My preventive program has helped so many people achieve a new level of confidence and oral health, with cleaner-feeling teeth, fresher breath, and fewer, happier dental visits. These are important achievements that have often elevated patient attitudes to dentistry—even for those who admit they once truly wished to *kiss their dentist goodbye.*

10

You and Your Dentist— Can You Ever Be Friends?

Friends are those rare people who ask how we are,
and then wait to hear the answer.

—EDWARD CUNNINGHAM, AMERICAN ENTREPRENEUR
AND AUTHOR OF *RECIPROCITY*

As this book has already established by now, you do *not* have to rely solely on a dentist to keep your mouth healthy. On the other hand, it is important to monitor all these dynamic changes in your oral health so you will be sure that it improves and then remains in great shape. Remember that *most* people either think they were "born" with good teeth, or that they somehow *deserve* to get cavities because they may have missed a dental cleaning or canceled an appointment. Through a series of perpetuated narratives, dentistry continues to offer its own misleading "myths"—many of which have caused patients to feel all manner of unnecessary guilt, worry, or fear. Those days are over—it's time for you to STOP letting someone (even *yourself*) carry the burden of self-directed blame.

The strategies offered throughout this book are likely to be radically different from the advice you have been given by your dentist. Facts being facts, you now need to consider that although you may love your dentist, his or her dental school education was most likely built on what should be called a "drill and fill" approach to tooth care. New technology has certainly improved treatments—indeed, the field of dentistry now benefits from all manner of computer-generated cavity design, crowns, fillings, implants, and even "fit in one day" dentures. The travesty is that this restorative work only remains necessary because of damage caused by a disease—one that could have been halted by small changes in habits and healed naturally with correct strategies.

Most people have never considered the importance of taking responsibility for their own oral health—by reading this book, of course, you already recognize its value. You will quickly feel improvements and positive changes, but to move forward, you need your progress to be *truthfully* evaluated by a dentist who understands the bigger picture. Once you have scheduled a dental evaluation, prepare yourself to listen carefully during the appointment—and do your best to try to absorb and understand the *meaning* of the findings. In that way, you can ask questions and contribute to any discussions about treatments that you or your family may want or need. These action-based decisions could be about how often to go for assessment visits, which treatments to accept, and which ones you want either to delay—or to *refuse*.

To monitor your oral health, and to ensure you feel confident that you are headed in the right direction, you will need professional advice from a supportive dentist who will understand your side of any decision-making processes. My hope is that this chapter:

- Will help guide you to find such a dentist;

- Will steer you toward the kind of evaluation scenario that ensures better oral health;

- Will provide you with the best and most important questions to ask at an appointment;

- And, if necessary, will equip you with what to do if things are not working out between you and your dentist.

HOW TO FIND A DENTIST

Selecting a dentist takes effort and it is not easy, but it is arguably an even more important decision than the choice of contractor to renovate your home. Our mouth's "contractor"—yes, this is how we will refer to your dentist for the purpose of this example—has the power to help you enjoy a lifetime of sustainable mouth health . . . or to precipitate an opposite sequence of calamitous events. A builder who doesn't care about the quality of the materials used, or the way they are applied, is more than partially responsible for structural flaws that may occur over the years to cause a house to slowly crumble and fall.

Underlying problems created by poor dental treatments can be hidden for years, but their long-term health effects are now being recognized as more serious than we previously imagined. Inferior or *toxic* dental materials can have a negative impact on overall health, and chronically infected teeth or gums can cause potential damage to our heart, body, and brain—outcomes that may only become obvious later in life, when it is too late to turn back the clock.

Dentists have different ways of treating patients. At this point, most oral health professionals still subscribe to the training and practice protocols espoused by the American Dental Association (ADA)—which is to say a non-personalized, "one size fits all" approach to dentistry. These dentists will ordinarily take charge of your situation, "drill or fill" your teeth to get you out of any painful circumstance, and then work over some period of time to make your teeth as functional as possible—for as *long* as possible. Their goal is not to save you from treatment—instead, it is to make your mouth comfortable so that you can go about your life and be able to eat and chew without too much harm or fuss.

This is the kind of dentistry that most people have requested—or is what they believe to be the only *plausible* kind that is available to them and their family. Today, many dentists operate their offices under the umbrella of far larger business corporations—ones that frequently possess allied and interconnected associations with dental insurance companies. These "big box" dental chains are always busy by design and are specifically appointed to do as much restorative dental work as possible. Because *more* is their motto, you should *not* expect them to favor—or want to treat—anyone who wants the least treatment possible.

On the opposite side of the spectrum are oral health professionals who are not trained in a specific dental specialty, but they choose not to follow the routine practice protocol of the American Dental Association (ADA). These dentists have usually attended training courses in methods for the "safe" removal of silver amalgam fillings with techniques, equipment, and even protective clothing to shield patients and staff from any toxicity during a filling—something that is generally not a concern for mainstream dentistry. Patients may also be offered intravenous and supplemental vitamins as support during treatment, and biological dentists promote far more personalized and holistic (or "whole-body") care.

Biological dentists are also sometimes referred to as "natural" dentists, yet surprisingly their offices are usually extremely busy with the removal and replacement of *all* the silver amalgam fillings you may have in *any* of your teeth. They disapprove of fluoride and reject any fluoride-containing oral care products, which is why I believe that the guidance of a biologic dentist can frequently lead clients to require ongoing treatment and an incessant need for fillings to be repeatedly and frequently replaced, often culminating in the eventual *death* of these over-treated teeth. The biological practitioner treatment choice for a dead tooth is usually to extract it, since they also believe that root canals are unsafe. This means biological dentists also do a lot of implants, bone grafting, and other surgeries, and patients can spend thousands of dollars for an elegant *style* of treatment, yet the outcome often does not reflect a naturally healthy mouth and minimal treatment that I believe is both possible and *ideal*.

So, which kind of dentist do you want? Everyone needs a dentist who values pristine (*uncut*) teeth; who wants to avoid drilling, when possible; and one who has been trained in techniques of tooth repair that mimic the structure of nature's original design—through use of a minimally invasive approach. Most of us want to keep our own teeth in a healthy condition for life, with no unnecessary treatments. You may be lucky to have such a dentist—but if you are looking, you may gather some names from a group of specialized care professionals referred to as *biomimetic* dentists.

There are only a few such-trained dentists in America, with a smattering of others located elsewhere around the world. These biomimetic dentists spend hours learning specialized techniques to correctly fill teeth with fiberglass materials, all of which help to care for the overall integrity of your teeth. You may not find one near your home, but perhaps you can find one in a city you visit, or at a vacation spot where you could start with a comprehensive dental evaluation.

"BAD" DENTISTRY

There is no way for a patient to evaluate the techniques or materials being used during their dental treatment. Even if a dentist notices previously performed and shoddy dental work in your mouth, he or she may not divulge it to you. Too often, patients will accept the blame if food gets stuck between their teeth—something that may, in fact, result from one or more dental mistakes; a poorly shaped filling; or a roughness or ledge that can form if an edge of the filling does not align smoothly with the adjacent tooth surface.

Sometimes, a dentist may inadvertently cut an adjacent tooth surface with his drill and expose this area to decay by removing its protective enamel surface. These are accidental incidents that should never happen, but they do—and as an untrained layperson, you will likely never know or discover when or if they have happened to you. Fragments of fillings can end up in your mouth and be swallowed, especially as old fillings are removed, or when new ones are being put into teeth. Both silver and plastic particles can affect the health of your gut, as their toxins can damage gut bacteria or affect your hormones.

There are also times when a rough cleaning, an unnecessary crown, a retainer, or a poorly designed night guard can create long-term consequences that could be easily classified as "bad" dentistry. This is why you need a caring, thoughtful, and experienced dentist.

DENTAL ETHICS

The professional training and direct experiences of every dentist eventually combine—and when these are mixed with an individual's personality, it creates a unique approach to dental care. A dentist's career experience *matters*. Most who have spent time treating the elderly or patients with physical or mental disabilities; worked in clinics for the underserved; or in countries where dental equipment is not available will understand there is a realm beyond dental school and decision making in the real world that is different from the formulas and standard protocols they may have originally been taught. Integrity is doing what is right, even when there is no glory or money in the outcome. If you have an experienced dentist with integrity, be thankful and enjoy the benefits.

An American-trained pediatric dentist often has no practical experience between dental school and entering this field of specialization. This can narrow their long-term view and blur their selection of treatment choices for their young patients. For example, a dentist may not realize when treating a child how critical is her or his decision to drill a ten-year-old tooth, which can impact and potentially precipitate a lifetime of future treatment needs for this tooth. Why seal or drill if you could reverse this cavity and improve the oral health trajectory for this child? Traditional pediatric dentists may be satisfied with the look of nickel-metal crowns on root canal-treated teeth, plastic coatings, strong fluoride gels and sealants, done as the child is sedated by a general anesthetic. From a global perspective, however, this can seem barbaric, dangerous, and unnecessary—especially when there are other options.

A more compassionate kind of "no drill" dentistry is called an Atraumatic Restorative Technique (ART) approach, an effective and *respected* approach to children's dental treatment and care.

The ART Pediatric Approach

"ART" stands for Atraumatic Restorative Treatment, and it has been my personal choice as a valid approach to solving the problem of decay in children's teeth for decades. The use of *silver* and *fluoride* used together in a varnish that stops decay is used as a way of treating cavities in baby teeth, and it is gaining acceptance in America with entrepreneurial dentists who have bucked "the system" and refuse to give in to ridicule or dismissal.

Baby teeth are vulnerable to decay, and cavities in baby teeth do not reverse, as they do in adult teeth. Stopping decay is critical, and xylitol is useful, but if the cavity needs to be filled, ART dentistry helps to avoid the use of a dental drill and is structured to provide treatment without pain; that requires no hospital visits; and, in most cases, can be achieved during a ten-minute "in and out" low-cost visit that prevents ongoing dental damage.

This ART technique allows cavities to be gently cleaned with hand instruments and then varnished with a silver compound (*silver diamine*) mixed with fluoride (to stop the decay)—and finally topped with a glass type of filling (*glass ionomer*) that helps to seal up and fill the cavity. It has been evaluated extensively and used successfully in remote areas around the world where decay is an urgent concern and dental equipment is lacking: namely, in parts of Africa, Mexico, and a number of regions in South America.

It has *also* been endorsed by the World Health Organization (WHO) as an effective method for managing decay, while also preserving tooth structure. Furthermore, the International Caries Consensus Collaboration—a group of dental professionals from twelve (12) countries who review strategies for dealing with tooth decay and promote their opinions to dentists across the world—also recommend ART as a treatment option for decayed teeth.

It has not yet, however, been embraced by the American Academy of Pediatric Dentistry (AAPD). Instead, the AAPD endorses a style of treatment known as Interim Therapeutic Restorations (ITR). This technique exactly resembles the technique of ART—using hand instruments to clear the decay and the application of silver diamine fluoride and a glass filling—but the AAPD protests that this a temporary, and not a permanent, solution. Combined with the preventive use of xylitol and improved oral care, these temporary fillings may be all your child needs until new permanent teeth come into the mouth. Meanwhile, do not confuse this approach with the use of a plastic sealant—something heavily promoted by the AAPD, but which may not be useful or even *necessary*.

WHEN AN EVALUATION IS NEEDED

Once you are confident that you are able to manage your dental maintenance effectively at home, then you will likely wish to discontinue any unnecessary bi-annual cleanings. After all, you now know that these professional cleanings present no magical power to combat the daily damage that your teeth experience. Dental cleanings cannot *stop* cavities or gum disease, although it is correct that they help people—to *some* degree—who are unwilling to help themselves.

The problem with these visits is that many of us have been brainwashed by marketing messages through voicemail and text for so many years. As such, the majority of the public are easily persuaded that these cleanings are a vital component of oral care. The intention of these reminders may be a legitimate effort to get you to the dental office for an evaluation of your teeth and gums—but the question to ask is whether you actually *need* this "one size fits all" bi-annual cleaning.

Yes, everyone needs an in-depth check of their oral health periodically, but this does not necessarily involve (or it may go far beyond) those routine X-rays and the so-called dental cleaning. This is why I encourage you to find an ethical, caring, and knowledgeable dentist, rather than look for one who merely "takes your insurance."

PREPARE FOR YOUR DENTAL VISIT

To gain the most benefit from dental visits, you want to feel comfortable when you get ready to go to the appointment with your goal of as little treatment as possible. To achieve this, it is best to prepare *prior* to a dental visit and do your best to reverse as many potential problems as you can. In other words, work to improve your oral health *before* the visit. My special Complete Mouth Care System™ (see Chapter Six) may take a year or two to help heal your gums and spruce up your teeth, but even a few weeks can help you to create a better impression during your mouth examination. Taking these active steps prior to the time when you sit down in that dental chair will give you sharper focus and clarity when it comes to your next step(s).

What to Eat Before (and After) a Dental Visit

Obviously, you don't want to have food around your teeth as you go into a dental visit—and I suggest that the *best* time to use my system is *within a few hours* of your appointment. In Chapter Eight, we talked about how saliva health is improved by diet and digestive health. Consider this prior to your dental visit and let saliva that has been boosted by good foods play a part in enhancing the condition of your teeth and gums.

Eating certain foods are also useful prior to and following any X-rays that you receive, as they contain nutrients that help protect our body from possible radiation damage. Vitamin C-rich foods, like oranges and lemons, will help the nerves in your jaw to recover more quickly after an anesthetic-numbing injection, and many foods (again, described in Chapter Eight) serve to stimulate skin and gum healing—particularly if your mouth is sore after your visit.

The Best Time for a Dental Visit

The timing of your visit is also something to consider. Particles of tooth and debris are sprayed into the air above every dental chair as a dentist drills, or when the hygienist works to clean a patient's teeth. This invisible cloud floats in the air for about twenty-four (24) hours and, following treatment of multiple patients, the office air could carry considerable amounts of unwanted bacteria. This is why dental teams gear up with goggles, masks, and sometimes even shielded helmets to protect themselves from this potentially infectious spray.

You, however, are expected to lie down on the chair with your mouth open, which is why it is good if your dentist covers your mouth with a protective latex square sheet referred to as a *dental dam*. (If your dentist's office has a high-powered vacuum exhaust system to keep the air cleaner and try to purify it, so much the better.) I *also* suggest you wear protective glasses—and for examination appoint-ments when there is no way for you to shield your mouth, it is always a good idea to make an early morning appointment (ideally after a long weekend) when the circulated air in the treatment room has had time to settle.

Do You Even *Need* a Dental Cleaning?

Anyone who has used my system of care for a year should begin to reach the point when they no longer form plaque and do not need "routine" cleanings every six months. As you initially phase into my system, a little dead plaque may accumulate as dark deposits in nooks and crannies, and even on porous flat surfaces in some mouths, but they are more generally found in places that are difficult for you to clean. You may have used a brush that was too soft, or perhaps you were afraid to brush vigorously. A cleaning appointment can quickly deal with this superficial debris and prepare you for moving forward with less chance of this build up on your teeth. Some hygienists may be confused, but you should know that these surface shadows or stains do not reflect negatively on your mouth health—they occurred *because* your mouth became healthier.

After this debris has been cleaned off your teeth, you will be pleased with the way your teeth look and feel because this was simply "left-over" remnants from the unhealthy mouth you had before starting my system of care. Be sure to continue with this routine, but bear in mind that you may *also* need a new or better toothbrush, or to more actively target those stained areas on your teeth as the first step in your daily brushing routine. In the future, you can ask your dentist how often you *need* a cleaning—and it is perfectly acceptable to ask for the reasons *why*.

WHAT IS A DENTAL EVALUATION?

A dental evaluation is different from those old twice-a-year "check-ups" that have usually always taken place alongside those obligatory X-rays and routine cleanings. We have already discussed at length the connection between body and mouth health—and this is why your entire head, neck, and systemic health should be considered part of a good dental evaluation. Some dentists will take your blood pressure, examine the health of your carotid arteries, and do a thorough examination for an array of problems—for instance, looking for ulcerations, a misaligned bite, or any hint of oral cancer. Usually, an examination will begin with a check of the outside of your head and neck, then your mouth, and finally a visual examination of your gums and teeth, followed by necessary X-rays—and, finally, any tests and/or treatments that you may require or want.

A Head and Neck Evaluation

An experienced hygienist or dentist will perform a head and neck examination by massaging and feeling around your neck, face, and lower jaw. This is done to determine if you have enlarged salivary glands or *nodes* (small glandular masses), which could indicate inflammation draining from an infection or other problems in your mouth.

Visual and Tactile Evaluation

A *soft tissue examination* is performed to evaluate the texture and color of your tongue, the skin on the inside your mouth, and the area that stretches down further into your throat. The dental examiner may move your tongue to look underneath it, or on the sides—places where ulceration may be a sign of so-called *pathology*, something which could suggest the start of an oral cancer. This kind of screening is valuable every few years, at a frequency related to your personal risk—for example, you may need this annually if you smoke; vape; drink alcohol; are diabetic; have a dry mouth from disease or medications; have had radiation and/or chemotherapy; have been exposed to the herpes virus; or have a family history of head and neck cancer.

During the visual examination, a pointed dental probe called an *explorer* (a kind of thin, "L"-shaped instrument normally comprised of metal) is gently trailed over your teeth to determine if there are any rough areas—and this tactile assessment is then matched with the *visual* one. If all the tooth surfaces look and feel smooth and hard, this is a good sign.

TOOTH HEALTH EVALUATION

In the 1950s, it was common for dentists to force this sharp pointed explorer against the surface of teeth to search for so-called *sticky spots* that were believed to be the early onset of cavities. Every suspicious area was poked or probed to see if the sharp point could break the surface—something that was interpreted as a tooth in need of a filling.

By 1966, research indicated that these soft areas could heal themselves completely with correct care, and that a potential cavity could disappear if minerals went back into the area. Pushing a metal point into a weak spot on a tooth could make this repair more difficult—sometimes *impossible*.

In 1992, a study in *The Journal of Caries Research* reported on one hundred teeth that were examined with an explorer point—and were then found to have sticky spots. The teeth were extracted, cut open, and examined under a microscope to see if this diagnosis of a cavity was accurate. Only twenty-four (24) of the teeth had signs of decay, showing how unreliable the explorer is for finding a cavity.

Today, a dentist should only examine teeth with a blunted explorer and only to feel for rough areas, which should then be allowed to remineralize. No dental professional should ever push any kind of sharp or pointed instrument into a tooth or grooves on the surfaces of teeth to *test* their hardness. Change your dentist if he or she uses a "pointy" explorer in this inappropriate way.

A PERIODONTAL EVALUATION

A *periodontal* or gum health examination should technically be a continuation of this soft tissue evaluation. The goal is for your gums to be tight against your teeth with no bleeding, with a somewhat indented appearance that gives the surface an almost pin-pricked texture—which should be pink, rather than red, in color—and with no loose pockets of periodontal disease. This is a good time to listen to the dentist or hygienist's evaluation and the numbers that they report on your dental chart.

At the conclusion of this stage of your appointment, you can ask for a printed copy of these numbers, or you can simply write down in a small notebook which of your teeth have been diagnosed with problematic pockets. You need to know if the pockets are on the inside or outside surfaces of your teeth, so that you will be confident which areas you need to target with your home care.

BLEEDING GUMS

Your hygienist may find an area that bleeds during his or her examination with a dental probe. This may happen if you are in the first months of improving your mouth health with my system. Bleeding is possible, even if you have worked hard to improve your oral health, and no matter if your mouth feels cleaner and healthier than ever before.

Some hygienists consider this a signal that you need to floss more frequently, but often the problem is caused by the fragile state of new gum tissue—like any wound in the process of healing. Perhaps you have not used the correct brushes, are not confident enough to do vigorous gum massage yet, or you forgot how important diet is for gum health. A little more work at home could likely resolve this so-called *bleeding on probing* (BOP)—so don't be dismayed, and maybe give yourself a few more months before re-evaluation.

GUM POCKETING

If areas of gum pocketing are discovered by your examiner, the depths of these pockets will be recorded in millimeter measurements at six separate spots around the root of *each* tooth. Ideally, you will want to know where any pockets are in your mouth, so you can target these specific spots with vigorous gum massage. As described in Chapter Six, my Complete Mouth Care System™ can usually help to heal pockets within six (6) to twelve (12) months, and you should expect to achieve zero pocketing around your natural teeth.

Be aware that implants cannot be evaluated with a probe in the same way as teeth, since there is no attachment of gums to an implant. Some hygienists probe implants, but there is disagreement about the usefulness of this. If pocket depths have improved since your last evaluation, even if a few continue to measure a few millimeters, try a few more months of slightly more focused gum massage; use good toothbrushes; ensure that you give your mouth more resting periods; and consider modifying your diet (strategies that were all explained in Chapter Eight).

Your dentist may offer laser treatments or deep cleaning to help reduce these gum pockets and remove any hardened debris found under the gums. This treatment may be helpful for some people, but the Complete Mouth Care System™ has allowed many to avoid this treatment and heal the associated pockets. This can even occur in situations where there is an accumulation of a crusty layer of plaque below the gum line. This so-called *tartar* or *calculus* can build into a sizeable plate of mineralized plaque, but the regular use of my suggested home care strategies can often dissolve it away—and gum massage can help resolve the pockets completely.

Never allow gum pocketing of more than seven (7) millimeters to linger more than a year—and if you have tried using my system for twelve (12) months and have not healed such a deep pocket by yourself, then a deep cleaning or surgery may be better for your mouth. In-office stem cell regenerative therapy is a way to promote gum and bone growth, in a similar fashion to the gum massage that I recommend. This treatment injects stem cells (see Chapter Eight for more on this topic) into your gums and uses lasers to excite these cells into a regrowth of healthy tissue in and around your gums. The outcome from this kind of therapy appears to be superior to other techniques that include bolstering the gums with collagen and dermal fillers or using bone and gum grafting.

GUM RECESSION

Gum recession can cause pain and tooth sensitivity, but it is not an indicator of poor mouth health. In fact, recession often occurs in healthy mouths from overuse of the wrong kinds of products (like baking soda, whitening pastes, or peroxide) or an excessive amount of flossing. This is why it is important to recognize the difference between gum disease (where you may need to do more) and gum recession (where you may need to do *less*). Knowing the *cause* of recession is important so it can be controlled—especially if you have enamel loss along the sides of your teeth, which makes it impossible for your gums to grow back across this empty (even-filled) enamel erosion space.

Filling the erosion grooves in enamel is often a recommendation, but if the area is temperature-sensitive, you may prefer to wait and use my system to reduce the sensitivity first, so you give the tooth time to protect the tooth nerves. This type of filling on the sides of teeth is called a *Class V (five)* filling, and they often fail and need constant replacement—which risks the health and vitality of these teeth. Ask your dentist *why* he or she recommends the filling of these eroded areas, and maybe discuss what he or she thinks about the idea of a delay in treatment.

Bacterial Testing

Cavities and gum disease are the result of an imbalance in the proportions of bacteria in your mouth. A sample of your saliva can be used to measure the number and kinds of mouth bacteria it contains, and also to help determine if you have an overabundance of harmful ones (periodontal pathogens or plaque-forming ones) or too few that are healthy (often a cause of bad breath).

How Often Do You Need X-Rays?

A visual inspection used to be the best way to judge the overall health of a mouth, but this is not possible if the biting surfaces of teeth have been sealed or filled. Molar grooves are usually the first places in the mouth to decay, which means we can make a relatively accurate interpretation that if someone has healthy molar grooves, they likely have a very healthy mouth. When these grooves are covered with a plastic sealant or have been otherwise masked or filled, then it must be understood that these treatments will have eradicated the most important signal for visual mouth assessment.

With an inability to check tooth groves, we can no longer rely on a visual examination and therefore need more frequent X-rays to monitor mouth health. This is another critical reason to avoid sealants and unnecessary fillings, since they considerably increase your lifetime need for—and dependence on—X-rays. The more dental work in your mouth, the more you will need X-rays—and the less fillings, crowns, bridgework, sealants, and implants that you have, the less X-rays you will need.

X-Rays for Evaluation of Progress

X-rays are also useful to find unexpected things, to determine if your teeth and jawbone look healthy and normal, and to investigate the ongoing health of specific areas. However, X-rays can also be a tool to show if your mouth care routine has successfully mineralized your teeth. When X-rays are aimed at a mineralized surface, they bounce off minerals they encounter—and the more X-rays bounce back, the whiter this area appears in an X-ray picture.

Examine an X-ray of a tooth and you will see that it has a white outer shell. When you compare X-rays taken from the same angle, targeted at the same tooth, and after an interval of time, it is possible to compare the brightness of this shell. Every year—if your teeth are in fact becoming healthier and more mineralized—this area of your teeth should look clearer and whiter. A dark area on an X-ray means this area is not mineralized, because there are no minerals to bounce the X-rays back. The center of a tooth always appears black because it is an empty space full of liquids, nerves, and live cells. The *dentin* of the tooth (see Chapter Two earlier in this book for more on this topic) has a few minerals, so it always appears as gray in color.

If your dentist sees a black shape in part of a tooth that is supposed to be gray or white, this indicates that there may be a loss of minerals in this area. These black shapes on an X-ray can easily look like a hole in your tooth, but this is not necessarily the case. A cavity takes some years to form, and it begins as a softened area where minerals have disappeared. If you decide to remineralize your teeth, then this black hole will likely brighten and whiten in color. Bear in mind that it can take months for a demineralized area to show up as fully mineralized on an X-ray. Improvement should be encouraging, and if you see progress, you should continue for longer to see if you can completely reverse this loss of minerals.

Bitewing X-rays are still the best type to show this kind of change, both in tooth density and mineralization. If your dentist needs to look closely at the area around the root of a tooth, he or she may take a *periapical* X-ray to see this unique view. A periapical X-ray can also be used to help determine if a tooth is dead or alive. More expansive and complete jaw X-rays are called *panoramic* X-rays, and they capture an image of your entire jaw—upper and lower—on one piece of film. This helps a dentist notice things that are unusual—a cyst, a buried or extra tooth, a left-over root from some previous extraction—or anything else that would be considered unexpected in the jaw area of the mouth.

Sometimes a dentist will use a panoramic X-ray to check the carotid artery blood vessels in your neck, if only to more fully ensure that there are no signs of a calcification blockage inside the walls of these arteries (which would appear on the X-ray as a white area or calcified mass). Other dentists may offer *ultrasonic scans* of these arteries—to similarly check the health of this important blood vessel that takes blood through your neck and into your brain. *Cone Beam Computed Tomography* (CT) scans are now used more commonly in dental offices. They are less expensive for the dentist, are said to create less radiation exposure, and can produce improved 3D images to help your dentist better evaluate the position and health of tooth roots or possible fractures. Fortunately, technologies are being developed to make no-radiation scans a possibility in the near future.

UNNECESSARY TREATMENTS

You need a dentist who will talk with you and explain how you could improve your oral health at home. In the summer of 2006, the *New York State Dental Journal* published an editorial examining the "biological price" of fillings, compared with the option of no treatment—that is, the comparison between the cost to health created or caused by a filling (in the form of possible harm to the mouth and body, and the potential risk for a filling to precipitate a cascade of future treatment requirements) compared with an outcome achieved by stabilization of mouth health if the patient chooses to reverse this cavity (which could potentially eliminate any need for a filling).

Consider carefully that some dentists do not believe that cavities or gum disease are preventable or reversible. You should also remain aware that there is another available treatment that flows a thin plastic sealant material into the open porosities of a cavity. This is *not* a good solution, since it can act as a kind of plaque magnet to attract decay in this area of the mouth—so don't be fooled by this sealant treatment for early cavities.

We have already explored how a small cavity in a permanent adult tooth can naturally reverse in a few months, which is why any motivated patient should weigh the risks of sealants and "small" fillings, and consider carefully that any treatment will be irreversible, especially if you allow a tooth to be randomly drilled. Patients often want to have a conversation with their dentist and be given options—including a non-treatment choice. Why put a filling into a tooth that could repair itself naturally? This is a question that *must* be asked, especially when this is a choice for young patients.

Toxicity of White Fillings and Sealants

Statistics show that more than fifty percent (50%) of silver amalgam fillings eventually need repair, and that the lifespan of an amalgam or white filling is about thirteen (13) years. Consider how many times one filling could be repaired over a lifetime and multiply this by the number of teeth in your mouth. There is always some damage and danger to the life of a tooth when a dentist removes or puts in fillings. Remember as well that there is always some impact from almost *all* dental materials, as mercury can escape from silver amalgams and plastic chemicals can leach from sealants and white fillings.

This is why I suggest you consider carefully if your dentist suggests that you change your silver fillings to white ones. White fillings attract plaque and can quickly develop cavities around their edges. All filling replacements have the potential to kill the nerve of a tooth, although this damage may occur slowly and not be obvious for five or more years. The fact that many teeth die and need a root canal after an amalgam has been replaced by plastic makes this replacement decision important.

White fillings and sealants are materials with ingredients that have the potential to cause what is called a *bisphenol toxicity*, which is a reaction that occurs when plastic molecules (with a specific chemical structure) are absorbed by the body or swallowed into the digestive tract. These chemicals confuse the body signaling systems as they mimic the important female cycle and growth regulating hormone called *estrogen*, and this can raise the overall impact and effects of estrogen everywhere in the body.

These toxic side effects could be a serious issue for a child or someone of reproductive age, or if you have a history of hormonal dysfunction or estrogen-related cancer in your family. You have been empowered by the material in this book to refuse unnecessary fillings, and you would do well to always remember the option to delay and wait for confirmation of the safety of white fillings and sealants on the gut microbiome—especially for children, young adults, and women of all ages.

Toxicity of Silver Fillings and Gum Disease

Silver amalgam fillings are banned in Norway, Denmark and Sweden, and many dentists in America refuse to use this material in their offices. The International Academy of Oral Medicine and Toxicology has established safety guidelines for the drilling and removal of amalgam fillings, and there are many dentists who offer the safe replacement of amalgam fillings, removing most of the danger posed by amalgam toxicity. I encourage patients to protect their existing fillings and maybe wait before they decide to exchange a silver filling for a white one, since in a healthy mouth, silver and white fillings should remain stable for life. If you are worried about toxicity, know that our body has many ways to detoxify and remove the poisons from dental materials, but the first way is to avoid any more fillings that would add to the toxic burden on the body.

On the other hand, it is vital to know that certain gum disease bacteria can release *hydrogen sulfide*—a gas that reacts with mercury (the compound that is found in silver amalgam fillings). When this gas reacts with the mercury from fillings, it can form a toxic compound called *mercuric sulfide*. If you have amalgam fillings in your mouth, it would be wise to take a salivary test and be assured that you do not have high levels of periodontal pathogens or chronic periodontal disease, since this has the potential for the formation of a highly toxic compound, which if released into your mouth has the potential to cause kidney and nervous system damage—if mercuric sulfide is absorbed or inhaled. A metallic taste in your mouth is a sign of this problem, and my recommendation is to immediately start using my system of care to reverse periodontal disease as rapidly as possible.

Smile Design

People want attractive teeth and although a nice smile is definitely a beauty asset, the alignment and color of your teeth does not define your mouth health. Front teeth are visible to others, and there is an interesting but illusionary line (created by the contrast in color between the white of your teeth and the pink of your lips) that creates your *smile line*. Look in a mirror and follow the tips of your upper teeth from the front to the tip of your last visible tooth when you smile. This smile line shape affects how others perceive your smile, with a gently upward-curved line associated with a wide, friendly smile.

If you now want to enhance your smile, there are specialists in cosmetic dentistry, prosthodontics, and orthodontics who suggest a variety of ways to build with crowns, veneers, bridges, or implants, or move teeth with orthodontic appliances to formulate a new smile. This is not easy to achieve so be cautious of online marketing that promotes "do it yourself" tooth movements—this is one case when you must have expert advice from an experienced specialist to move teeth safely.

One consequence of incorrect tooth movement is that gums can move down the roots—a problem we call receding gums. The way teeth bite together matters for the health of the gums and bone. If your teeth have been incorrectly moved, it can have long-term effects on your gums—and this can lead to eventual tooth loss and leave teeth without an appropriate bite, which could compromise your oral health for life. Before you worry about straightening your teeth, ensure your mouth is healthy. You will notice that a healthy smile naturally appears brighter and more attractive, anyway.

WHAT TO DO WHEN THINGS ARE NOT WORKING OUT

How do you find a dentist with high standards and who values teeth? The best dentist is surely one who does an ever-diminishing amount of work on your teeth. My advice is to be cautious and realize that descriptions can themselves be a marketing strategy. Many new dentists consider selecting a field of dentistry that will maximize their work goals, which may not be *your* goals. Cosmetic skills and whitening, or the idea of being holistic, are some of the strategies to set dental offices apart.

You may simply want an honest evaluation by a caring professional but even when you find such a dentist, be aware that there may still be some difficulties to overcome. You cannot change dental offices every time you and your dentist disagree, so I encourage you to be empowered with as much understanding of oral health as possible. You should ask questions and take your time to agree on any treatment plan. Below are some of the decisions that you may find easier with a little more knowledge.

Ten Ways to Empower Yourself Before a Dentist Visit

It is one thing to learn about all the best and most proactive things one should do for your teeth and gums in between dental visits—it is something else *entirely* when it comes to being—and *feeling*—adequately prepared for that next scheduled appointment. The following are ten surefire ideas you may want to consider before you go to your next dental visit.

1. Confidence can help you glide through a dental appointment, which is why you will want to take headphones and some favorite music. But you also want your teeth to look as good as possible, so know mouth health *can improve* in a few weeks and be sure to clean your teeth immediately before your scheduled visit.

2. Resist pressure or coercion by dental office staff who may suggest you should whiten your teeth. Bleaching treatments weaken teeth and ultimately make them more porous, so they will stain more easily if you decide to stop using whitening products. Improve your *daily home care* to *naturally* whiten your smile.

3. You may be told that you need dental work, or that your gums are not healthy. Don't allow this to make you sad or anxious. Avoid signing treatment agreements quickly, unless your problem is an emergency. You may want to consider options—even the option to reverse a cavity or gum disease yourself—or see a specialist for a second opinion. These are *your* teeth, and you do not need to commit to anything you do not *want* to have done—especially in a hurry.

4. You may not want to buy the products that your dentist recommends. *Never* allow yourself to feel pressured or purchase an expensive toothbrush or other device when there may be equally or *more* effective—and less expensive– options.

5. Knowledge is power, so I encourage patients to ask lots of questions at dental visits. A patient's responsibility is to provide the dentist with a good medical history and as much information as possible about any dental symptoms. Then be sure to listen and ask more questions if you do not understand your dentist's evaluation of your

teeth. You may want to know more about your periodontal charting and the urgency for treatment. With a clear picture you can be in a better position to decide what *you* want your dentist to do in *your* mouth.

6. Dentists may recommend that you, or your child, be referred to a specialist—maybe an orthodontist who specializes in straightening teeth, or an endodontist who specializes in evaluating sensitive teeth and has the skills to do a root canal on a dead tooth. This may be a good idea, but always take time to consider if you want to accept the procedures recommended and ensure you understand which treatments can *wait* and which ones should begin *immediately*.

7. If you are told that you have a small cavity or two, you can ask if it is possible to delay treatment for a few months. You can use my strategies and ask if they see improvement at your next appointment. Cavities generally take several years to form, and many cavities can be reversed—often within ten to twelve months. You may amaze your dentist when your improved oral care is able to heal those cavities.

8. A good time to take charge of oral health and make changes is *before* your next dental appointment. Mouth health can improve rapidly and make your teeth cleaner and healthier—especially when you use the strategies introduced in this book. If you need a dental cleaning, you will have less plaque—and if you need a filling, the tooth enamel will be stronger because of your efforts, so this new filling will be surrounded by healthier enamel and last longer in your mouth.

9. The air in most dental offices is contaminated by particles that spray out of mouths as teeth are drilled and cleaned. Your dental team wear masks and eye protection, but you lie in the chair with your mouth open. The best time for a dental appointment is early in the day—so you are the first in the treatment chair—ideally, after a long weekend (when the air has settled).

10. Last, if you take your child or children to the dentist, be sure to give them support by discussing and providing them with the same empowerment strategies listed above. They will thank you for it later.

Should You Extract a Tooth?

If a tooth nerve dies, what should you do? Some dentists tell you to extract the tooth, while others may advise you to have the tooth treated with a root canal. If you extract the tooth, you may find your dentist wants to make a bridge to fill the gap, while others suggest bone replacement surgery and an implant (which is a screw that carries a fake tooth). Extraction of any tooth is serious business, because there may be other options and health implications to consider. Extractions, even for children, is an option that should be weighed with the utmost of care. It is usually best, whenever possible, to save teeth rather than extract them too quickly—even if a smile is crowded—because there are a number of things about teeth that you may not know.

There are special nerve connections between adult teeth and the brain that cause the release of a substance called *orexin*, which may be a benefit for eye, digestive, and brain health. This is one good reason to try and save every possible tooth—including wisdom teeth. The jawbone around wisdom teeth will only grow to accommodate the tooth *if* there is one there—and although it may look as if there will never be room, consider waiting if your child has a healthy mouth and good oral care habits. If a tooth is extracted, the jawbone *will* stop growing, and this can shorten the jawbone and potentially impact the shape of a face and the size of nasal sinuses—which could impact breathing efficiency in later life. It is therefore crucial that you do not have any teeth extracted—unless there is an associated acute infection or tooth abscess, without the clear-minded consideration of these long-term effects.

Extractions themselves can be complicated, with serious potential to cause chronic nerve damage or a loss of taste or feeling in the tongue or lower jaw. A lost tooth creates a space, and if an upper tooth loses contact with its opposing lower tooth, this can allow the upper tooth to overgrow—and come loose—from the upper jaw. Implants also have drawbacks, while root canals have experienced a considerable amount of bad publicity on social media.

Implants are frequently sold as an easy dental fix, but they are *always* at high risk for periodontal gum disease—although when this so-called *periodontitis* infection is discovered around an implant, it is called *implantitis*. This is why it is so important to develop a healthy mouth *before* an implant.

Regular dental cleanings are also riskier for people with implants, as particles of titanium from the screw can be shaved off by hygiene instrumentation and cause tissue reactions that are similar in nature—and impact—to an exaggerated auto-immune response. If you already have implants yet continue to need dental cleanings, you may want to ask your hygienist if she or he will use what is referred to in the oral health industry as a special dental implant scaler to avoid this kind of implant scratching or possible complications.

So how can one decide the best dental treatment to select? In view of all these choices and considerations, my advice is to empower yourself with as much knowledge as possible—and to always seek out counsel, or at least a second opinion, from a specialist like an endodontist or prosthodontist.

THE STATUS QUO

Your dentist may tell you to use a soft brush and to avoid brushing your gums, but my recommendation is to practice consistent gum massage with a dense and relatively firm-textured brush. Some dentists say cavities cannot be reversed, but this book has suggested already how to do this. You may wish dentists would agree, but this is unlikely to happen in the foreseeable future.

Why? Well, a big part of the answer is because most are trained in the aforementioned "drill and fill" approach that fits the protocol structure of most dental offices, whereas you are now looking for personalized home care to avoid unnecessary dental treatments.

Unfortunately, financial reimbursement generally maintains the status quo in America, and student training is to fit the paradigm where dentists are paid a fee for service—and this means that the more treatment a dentist does for you, the more he or she is compensated with money. If your dentist has never seen a cavity reverse, then she or he will unfortunately be unable to offer you the kind of support that you now seek. If your dentist does not believe periodontal disease can be reversed without a cleaning, then *you* may need to consider following my protocol for a few months before you return.

Remember something, as you continue on this oral health journey: Your mouth's environmental conditions *cannot* go in two directions at the same time. If your teeth and gums feel cleaner and healthier, then keep going with my Complete Mouth Care System™. If you see some surface stains on your teeth, they are likely superficial and may even be successfully brushed away with a little more vigor. Don't make the mistake, though, of interpreting a temporary cosmetic flaw—which can easily be cleaned away by your dentist—as something to worry or redirect you. It is *not* the sign of a problem—rather, it indicates that plaque is being addressed and that your oral health is changing and now going in the right direction.

No Instant Decisions

Second opinions can be useful, and it is always best to try not to feel pressured or make any instant decisions. You should *never* give your consent to a treatment plan until you have had the time to consider it—*carefully*. If you are told that you need a cleaning or surgery, find out as much as possible about it and perhaps ask how long you could responsibly delay this appointment. Remember the story of journalist Helen Rumbelow (see Chapter Four), who defied warnings and achieved amazing improvement in her oral health? Your dentist may have been trained to believe the only solution for periodontal disease is achieved through antibiotics and cleanings. The problem is that these repeated deep cleanings may not solve your problems, and they have been shown to carry a special risk for *anyone* with gum disease.

Consider the following: Gum disease may increase your risk for an ischemic stroke, and the more severe the periodontal disease in your mouth, the higher this risk appears to be, particularly for young adults. The *Journal of Dental Research* published the results of an international, multicenter study in April 2024 that investigated 348 people with periodontal disease and how their risk for stroke increased after a deep cleaning. This case-controlled study of adults ages 18 to 49 years old compared the experiences of first-ever stroke victims who had a Cryptogenic Ischemic Stroke (CIS), and this group was matched with adults of similar sex and age who were stroke-free. Invasive dental treatments, like deep dental cleanings three months prior, were found to be associated *significantly* with an increased risk for stroke. The participants in this study were recruited at Helsinki and Turku University Hospitals between 2013 and 2019 and it appears more studies are necessary to better understand these risks and dangers.

My suggestion, if you are diagnosed with gum disease, is to ask if your dentist would at least *consider* a delay. You can then look to make immediate use of my Complete Mouth Care System™, if only for a few weeks, to try and improve your oral health and limit this risk on your own—*prior* to a deep cleaning appointment.

CONCLUSION

At this moment, you may be ready to adopt the strategies in this book, even before your next visit, or maybe you are too nervous to do things that are contrary to the advice you have been given by your dentist. If you feel this way, or simply want to learn more, I have already created a number of online videos, teaching programs, and video interviews with dentists, doctors, and scientists where we discuss this new paradigm of dentistry, in a way that I hope will make you feel more comfortable and confident.

One vital nugget that I hope you have taken from these chapters is that oral health success *is possible*. Although the ideal moment to start using these strategies is *before* or *between* visits, it is *never* too late—and remember that most of these positive changes will occur largely in the comfort of your own home.

Don't buy into the excuse that you have a "cracked" tooth, or that your teeth are "aging," or the idea that you cannot control dental damage and must resign yourself to ongoing dental treatments. If you have any dental problems, immediately consider a change to your daily home care since healthy enamel does not crack, and a healthy mouth preserves fillings so that they do not age. You already know how to turn your mouth health around *before* your dentist makes that crown or refills that tooth. You have learned the power of stem cells and the process of *angiogenesis* to repair gum and bone, and how diligence with the Complete Mouth Care System™ can help you to reverse dental problems. The ideal is to prevent dental disease early in life and establish healthy habits in children so that they can enjoy a lifetime of perfect teeth.

I have always worked to help patients improve the quality of their dental visits. To do this, you must know how to control mouth health and how to avoid unnecessary treatments. My hope is that you have been empowered by this book and that you are now ready to enjoy your own future dental experiences—more than you may ever have believed possible.

Conclusion

All truth passes through three stages: first it is ridiculed, second it is violently opposed, and third it is accepted as self-evident.

—Arthur Schopenhauer, nineteenth-century philosopher

The medical and dental professions of today do not seem adequately aware of the simple things that patients can do for themselves to avert dental disease and suffering. This is why I believe it is important for patients themselves to be empowered about the dangers of commonly offered procedures like sealing tooth grooves, artificial tooth whitening, implants, and inappropriate straightening of teeth. Your body health, cognition, and longevity depend on interactions with your teeth and a healthy mouth. Powerful dental organizations seem focused on their financial stakes, while teaching institutions prepare dentists for general practice without concern for the long-term consequences of unnecessary treatments.

This is why I wanted to demystify oral biochemistry—and help you learn how to heal and strengthen your teeth with simple at-home strategies. My deep hope is that this book has served that purpose for you. In fact, nothing would put a bigger smile on my face than knowing that *Kiss Your Dentist Goodbye* has refreshed your mindset about dentistry, improved your oral health, and offered tangible nuggets of encouragement. For all who have dared to take a healthy bite into this book, I congratulate and thank you.

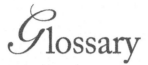

Glossary

Abrasion. The wearing away or loss of tooth enamel that occurs when the mouth is acidic, when teeth have inadequate lubrication and protection from mouth's liquids (dry mouth), and a signal to dentists to investigate for an underlying airway/breathing problem.

Aggregatibacter actinomycetemcomitans **(AA).** A type of bacteria that proliferates in mouth conditions associated with periodontal gum disease. AA is also associated with chronic sinus infections, and the bacteria can enter the bloodstream to negatively impact body health by evading and attacking immune cells.

Amalgam. A silver-colored metal material used to fill cavities in teeth. Half of the material is liquid mercury mixed with powdered silver, tin, and copper metals. Concerns about mercury toxicity have eroded its popularity, and many dentists use plastic or ceramic as filling materials instead.

Ameloblasts. These special cells are involved in a complex process that results in tooth formation inside the jawbone—before teeth enter the mouth. These cells release proteins and minerals that mix to create an enamel shell on the outermost part of a tooth.

Anaerobic. This refers to organisms that can exist in the absence of oxygen.

Angiogenesis. A process by which new blood vessels form from pre-existing ones, something that plays a vital part in wound and gum healing. The new vessels bring blood, oxygen, nutrients, and stem cells to support and accelerate the natural repair mechanism.

Biofilm. A community of resistant bacteria that adhere to surfaces and create a self-produced protective matrix, usually made from simple sugars called *polysaccharides* and *proteins* and with the inclusion of other bacteria.

Biomarker(s). Substances in blood that can be used to measure body reactions to medical interventions.

Biome. A diverse community of organisms in specific locations on or inside the body and comprised of bacteria, viruses, fungi, and other microbes. The composition can be shaped by diet, lifestyle, genetics, and interactions between bacteria. (See also *Microbiome.*)

Bisphenol toxicity. Harmful endocrine-disrupting effects associated with exposure to chemicals in plastics and resins, including white dental fillings and sealants. The most well-known is bisphenol A (BPA) toxicity, but there are variants called Bisphenol S (BPS) and Bisphenol F (BPF) that also block or mimic hormones (particularly estrogen) and create a range of adverse effects on reproductive, neurological, cardiovascular, and immune health, which may promote cancer and metabolic conditions such as obesity, and type 2 diabetes, and impaired glucose metabolism.

Brachiocephalic vein. A large vein found on the left and right side of the head that collects oxygen-depleted blood from the head, neck, arms, and upper chest to channel into the heart for re-oxygenation in the lungs.

Bruxism. An involuntary grinding or clenching of teeth during the day (or night) that causes tooth wear and damage, jaw pain, headaches, and loss of gum attachment. A serious underlying cause may be some kind of restriction in the airway from the nose or mouth into the lungs.

Butyrate. Also known as *butyric acid,* this is a beneficial compound essential to maintain the integrity of the gut lining that may help to prevent a condition called "leaky gut." (See also *Intestinal permeability* and *Leaky gut syndrome.*)

Calcium. A mineral that is essential for building and maintaining strong bones and teeth, but it also plays a key role in muscle, nerve, blood and overall body health.

Calculus. (See *Tartar.*)

Canine (tooth). A pointed, cone-shape tooth at the corner of the upper and lower jaws and located directly under the eyes (which is why they are sometimes called "eye teeth"). These strong teeth guide others into the mouth and provide support for our face and lips.

Capillaries. Small blood vessels that form a network that connects the body's oxygenated blood vessels with the blood vessels carrying deoxygenated blood back to the heart. They allow for the exchange of oxygen, nutrients, and other products between the blood and tissues at every location around the body.

Carotid artery. A major blood vessel that supplies oxygenated blood to the brain, face, and head, running up each side of the neck to further supply the outer parts of the head and the deeper parts of the brain, eye, and other areas in the skull. Carotid artery health is vital, and plaque build-up in carotid arteries can reduce blood flow and increase the risk for stroke.

Cariostatic. A substance or action that can halt or inhibit the development of tooth decay (*dental caries*).

Catalyst. A substance or other similar agent that provokes or speeds a reaction or change in the body.

Cavity. A damaged area of a tooth that is formed by the caving in of its structure, following the progressive weakening and erosion that results from the acidic attack of plaque bacteria.

Chlorine-dioxide. A solution used to sanitize food and produce. In mouthwash, it can disrupt anaerobic bacteria without producing harmful byproducts.

Circadian rhythm. A natural process that cycles over a period of twenty-four (24) hours. The rhythm can be influenced by environmental factors, hormones, and lifestyle, and related disruptions can then lead to health imbalances.

Citric acid. An organic acid found in citrus fruits like lemons, limes, and oranges, and which has a sour taste. It is used to flavor foods and beverages but can also play a part in the body's metabolism to create energy in our cells.

Collagen. A protein that provides strength, structure, and resilience to body tissues, including the gums and teeth. Collagen also forms attachment points where fibers connect the tooth to the jawbone and is also a *part* of these same attachment fibers.

Colonization. The process by which bacteria establish themselves to become stable communities suited to a particular environment within the body.

Crown. Dental crowns cover damaged, decayed, or unattractive teeth to restore function and their appearance—or to protect weak teeth from further damage. A crown is made by shaving away the outside layer of a tooth and replacing it with either metal, ceramic, porcelain, or plastic.

Curcumin. The root (or *rhizome*) of the South Asian plant called *Curcuma longa* provides a yellow-orange spice called *turmeric*, which is used in cooking and for medicinal purposes. The active compound in turmeric is *curcumin*, which has powerful anti-inflammatory and antioxidant properties.

Demineralization. A loss of minerals, which weakens a tooth's structure.

Dental caries. A progressive and destructive disease that attacks teeth.

Dentin. A porous, creamy white layer that is the principal mass of a tooth, within an outer protective layer and encasing live tissue in the center.

Dilute. The process whereby particles in a liquid become spaced out as more liquid is added. Since the thickness of a substance decreases by adding liquid, this process of dilution then makes the substance less concentrated and "weaker."

Electrolyte. A substance that, when dissolved in a liquid, can conduct electricity. Electrolytes are involved in many bodily functions, as they help to regulate water distribution and balance the fluids inside and outside our cells. They also play a role in nerve and muscle function.

Enamel. The hard outside layer of a tooth, packed with minerals to form a protective coating.

Endodontist. A dentist with additional training to diagnose and treat problems that occur on the inside live part of a tooth. These experts perform root canal treatments that can allow you to save a tooth from extraction.

Enzyme. Since our body needs certain proteins to speed chemical reactions—especially for digestion and wound repair—enzymes have a shape that allows them to attach to molecules, which thereby helps to achieve the process. For example, *amylase* (a mouth enzyme) speeds the breakdown of starchy foods into digestible sugars.

Erethism. A disorder that affects the nervous system and is often the result of long exposure to heavy metals and particularly mercury vapor. Symptoms include irritability, anxiety, loss of memory, hand tremors, and impaired brain function.

Erosion. The act of teeth wearing away, following a softening from prolonged exposure to acidity.

Essential oil(s). Highly concentrated extracts that release a plant's unique natural scent, flavor, and beneficial compounds. They can be made from various parts of a plant, including the leaves, flowers, stems, roots, or bark but they must be carefully diluted for use in any therapy or personal care product.

Estrogen. A sex hormone that plays a critical role in the regulation of the female reproductive system, influencing hormonal cycles and the development of a female body shape. This hormone is also important for bone, cardiovascular, and brain health—while imbalances of this hormone can lead to health deterioration in general (and cancer, in particular).

Eustachian tube(s). Each ear has a narrow tube connecting the middle ear to the throat. The function of this tube is to equalize air pressure on both sides of the eardrum for hearing and balance.

Explorer. A pointed instrument that dentists use to check for cavities and tooth decay.

Extraction. A procedure to remove a tooth from its socket—usually as a last resort when other treatments have failed or are not possible.

Filling(s). A dental treatment used when a tooth has been severely damaged by decay or fracture. A filling is designed to control dental pain and protect the tooth from further damage. White plastic and silver amalgam fillings are common, but ceramic/glass and gold are preferable.

Fluoridation. The process of adding extra fluoride to drinking water or oral care products, in an effort to strengthen teeth and help them resist decay. (See also *Fluoride* and *Fluorosis*.)

Fluoride. Fluoride is a mineral found in soil, water, and certain foods (such as brewed teas, along with certain fruits, vegetables, and fish) around the world. (See also *Fluoridation* and *Fluorosis*.)

Fluorosis. Mottling of the teeth caused by fluoride as it interferes with enamel formation in a child before the age of six, to result in a speckled or mottled appearance of enamel. (See also *Fluoridation* and *Fluoride*.)

Floss (Flossing). A thin strand of material promoted for cleaning teeth by rubbing it between teeth to remove stuck food particles.

***Fusobacterium* bacteria.** Rod-shaped bacteria that thrive in low-oxygen conditions found in the gut, breathing tubes, genital areas, and the gums around teeth. These bacteria can invade the body and may be involved in colorectal cancer.

Gingivectomy. A procedure that cuts gum tissues around teeth in an effort to make it easier for someone to clean their gums.

Gingivitis. A reversible inflammation of the gums most often noticed as "bleeding gums."

Glycerin (or Glycerol). A sweet, colorless, sugar alcohol commonly added to foods and cosmetics to help them retains moisture. Glycerin is derived from animal and plant fats by hydrolysis, and some from petroleum.

Graft. A surgical procedure that takes skin from one area and attaches it to another area where skin is needed. Gingival grafts are usually removed from the roof of the mouth and attached where gums are missing or receding.

Halitosis. A medical term for bad or "stinky" breath.

Human Papilloma Virus (HPV). A group of over 200 kinds of viruses, with some being able to infect the skin and mouth to cause warts or cancer. HPV is transmitted through skin-to-skin contact during sex, and these risks can be reduced by safer sexual practices and vaccinations.

Hydrogen peroxide. A chemical compound normally mixed with water to disinfect, bleach, and kill bacteria, viruses, and fungi. It can also change tooth color when used in artificial whitening products.

Hydroxyapatite (crystals). A naturally occurring mineral found in human bones and teeth, where it gives these structures strength and resilience.

Hygroscopic pull. Hygroscopic substances attract moisture from their surroundings, drawing or "pulling" water to themselves.

Implant. Used to replace a missing tooth, titanium or some biocompatible component is screwed into or attached to the jawbone, where it goes through a process of fusing with the bone. Once this has occurred the implant can support a replacement tooth.

Incisor. Eight thin, flat teeth that are located at the front of the mouth—four in the upper and four in the lower jaw. These teeth help us bite into food, and also help us talk and look friendly as we smile.

Interproximal cavity. Dental disease between two adjacent teeth occurs in a space known as an interdental or interproximal area. These cavities are often the result of microfractures in the enamel surface, that happen when biting forces are re-routed by a filling. Plaque bacteria enter the microfractures and begin to form a cavity.

Intestinal permeability. The ability for water and nutrients to pass through the intestinal walls into the bloodstream. When this permeability increases, it can allow other particles to pass through as well. When this occurs, it can cause leaky gut syndrome, potentially creating some gastrointestinal diseases. (See also *Butyrate* and *Leaky gut syndrome.*)

Invisalign®. A brand of transparent plastic and removable dental appliances used as an alternative to traditional metal braces. These aligners are customized using 3D-imaging technology to generate gradual tooth movements over a period of one to two years.

Knoop Hardness Test (KHT) and Knoop Hardness Number (KHN). This measurement was developed by Frederick Knoop at the National Bureau of Standards (now NIST) in 1939. A precise force is applied to the sample material by a diamond indenter with a specific shape. The material is examined under a microscope and the hardness number calculated from the result. This is a test used for brittle or thin materials, such as ceramics, glass and tooth enamel.

Lattice. Tooth enamel has a microscopic structure described as a lattice. It is a highly organized arrangement of crystals packed in a prism-like pattern, which gives enamel its remarkable strength and resilience.

Leaky gut syndrome. When too many substances are able to pass through the intestinal walls into your bloodstream, this may create a condition referred to as *leaky gut syndrome*. Symptoms may include aches and pains, bloating, cramps, gas, and sensitivity to certain foods. (See also *Butyrate* and *Intestinal permeability*.)

Lichen planus. A chronic condition that can affect the mouth, skin, nails, and sometimes the scalp. It is like an itchy rash and in the mouth may form white patches on the cheeks, gums, tongue and lips. Dental materials and medications can trigger the problem, which may have periods of flare ups and remission.

Litmus paper. Specially treated paper is used to measure acidity and record it as a pH number, by matching the color of the paper with a graded scale. The dyes in the paper change when they are exposed to different levels of acidity and the results are from pH 1 to 14, with a neutral pH registering as pH 7.

Lymph. A clear fluid that circulates in the body to help maintain fluid balance, remove waste, and support immune function.

Maltitol. A sugar alcohol derived from starches like corn. It is less sweet than table sugar and contains less calories. (It does *not* have the same oral health benefits as xylitol.)

Mannitol. A sugar alcohol that is naturally found in fruits and vegetables, including strawberries, mushrooms, and seaweed. It is a low-calorie sweetener commonly used in pharmaceutical products.

Mercury. A unique metal that is liquid at room temperature, with a silvery appearance. It has been widely used in dentistry and other industries, but its toxicity can have serious health and environmental impact.

Meta-analysis. A powerful tool for research to improve precision and accuracy in assessing study results by pooling data from multiple studies to look for patterns or trends that may not have been visible in individual studies. The reliability of meta-analysis depends on the quality of the studies and poor studies cause a bias in the results.

Metastable. A physical or chemical system that is temporarily stuck in an unstable condition, until something triggers its transition to become stabilized.

Microbiology. The scientific study of tiny, single-celled organisms that can only be seen under a microscope. These organisms include bacteria, viruses, fungi, and algae.

Microbiome. A diverse community of organisms living in a specific location on, or inside, the body. Every microbiome has a unique mix of bacteria, viruses, fungi and its composition is dynamic and shaped by factors such as diet, lifestyle, genetic traits, and other bacteria. (See also *Biome*.)

Microorganism. A living organism of microscopic size which makes it too small to be seen with the eye. Examples are bacteria, viruses, and fungi.

Miswak stick. A traditional, tooth-cleaning tool cut from twigs or roots of certain trees like the Salvadora persica—known as the "toothbrush tree." Miswak sticks contain silica, essential oils, and fluoride to offer antibacterial, plaque-removing, and teeth-whitening properties.

Moh's scale. A measure of mineral hardness generated by the ability of a mineral to scratch or be scratched by other substances. The scale ranks from 1 to 10 with 10 being the hardest, and enamel with a hardness of 5 and steel 4.5.

Nano-hydroxyapatite (NHA) toothpaste. A toothpaste that contains extremely small particles of hydroxyapatite minerals. The idea is these small particles fill microscopic cracks and block demineralized pores in the tooth enamel surface.

Neuropeptide. A small protein-like molecule that plays a crucial role in transmitting signals to the nervous system. Some neuropeptides help reduce the sensation of pain and others regulate stress, emotions, appetite, and the immune system. (See also *Orexin.*)

Night or mouth guards. Sometimes a guard is made to protect teeth from sports injuries, but more often they are made to protect teeth and jaw joints from wear and damage that causes pain and sensitivity after clenching and tooth grinding during sleep. The underlying cause of clenching and grinding may be a misaligned bite or an obstructed airway. This means night guards do not address the cause—which *should* be addressed.

Nitrate(s). Naturally occurring compounds found in foods, especially green leafy vegetables and in drinking water in agricultural areas where nitrogen-based fertilizers get into the water supplies.

Nitric oxide. In the body nitrates are converted to nitrites, which then form nitric oxide—a molecule that helps reduce blood pressure, and improve breathing, heart efficiency, and blood flow to the brain.

Nitrite(s). Chemical compounds that are known as food preservatives in cured meats, but they are also produced in the body by certain bacteria that live in the mouth.

Nitrous oxide. Commonly known as "laughing gas," this gas has been used in dentistry to relieve pain and for its mild sedative effects. When inhaled nitrous oxide creates a feeling of relaxation and reduces anxiety. The effects wear away rapidly as inhalation stops. Nitrous oxide has an environmental impact three hundred (300) times more potent than carbon dioxide.

Oligosaccharide. A complex carbohydrate found in vegetables, legumes, and grains. They provide energy to beneficial gut bacteria and support immune function.

Oral epithelium. A layer of cells that forms a covering over the lips, cheeks, gums, tongue, protecting these surfaces from mechanical, chemical, and bacterial attack.

Orexin. A substance (called a *neuropeptide*) secreted by the brain that affects and regulates wakefulness by its effects on our eyes, cognitive function, balance, and appetite. (See also *Neuropeptide*.)

Oropharyngeal cancer. Cancer found in the middle part of the throat, back of the tongue, or on the soft palate. It is often associated with smoking and alcohol consumption or following an HPV virus infection.

Otitis media. Inflammation in air-filled spaces behind the eardrum after a bacterial or virus infection that causes earache and fever—also known as a middle ear infection.

Pathogen. A kind of bacteria, virus, fungi, or parasite that can causes disease by invading the body and disrupting normal body functions.

Pentose. An important sugar that has a unique structure composed of five carbon atoms. These sugars are essential building blocks for DNA and RNA, and they are also involved in generating cellular energy, which is vital for cellular function. Xylitol is a pentose sugar. (See also *Xylitol*.)

Peptostreptococcus **bacteria.** An aggressive bacterium that thrives in low oxygen conditions and is often associated with infection in the mouth and nasal sinuses.

Periodontal disease. A more severe progression of gingivitis that occurs when the fibers of tooth attachment become infected and disrupted below the gum line.

Peroxide. (See *Hydrogen peroxide*.)

pH scale. A system to measure the acidity or alkalinity of a solution. The range is from zero (pH 0) to fourteen (pH 14), with seven (pH 7) being a neutral solution. Any number above seven is alkaline and any number below seven is acidic. The scale is designed so that each number represents a tenfold change in acidity: for example, a liquid with a pH of 3 is ten times more acidic than a solution with a pH of 4.

Phosphate. A chemical compound that is important for energy production in the body, to maintain the body's acid/alkaline balance, and for bone and tooth mineralization.

Phosphoric acid. Used in industry to produce fertilizers and remove rust, this acid is frequently used for its sour taste in a number of carbonated soft drinks. In dentistry, this acid is used to dissolve minerals from teeth and create microscopic holes in the enamel surface. Plastic can flow into these pores, and this is how the filling is attached to the tooth surface.

Planktonic (bacteria). Free floating bacteria that drift independently as opposed to existing inside surface biofilm, which makes them more susceptible to the effects of antiseptics and antibiotics than bacteria that are protected within biofilm.

Plaque. The soft sticky film that coats the teeth and contains bacteria. If left untreated, it can harden into tartar. (See also *Tartar.*)

Polyfluoroalkyl substances (PFAS). A group of industrial "forever" chemicals used for their resistance to water, oil and heat. They are used in non-stick cookware, many kinds of packaging and to make dental floss glide between teeth. These chemicals are toxic to the environment and can accumulate in the human body over time, being associated with hormone disruption, immune system impact, and a higher risk for cancer.

Polymerase Chain Reaction (PCR). This is a lab technique which can amplify parts of a DNA molecule to make billions of copies and allows scientists to perform genetic testing and disease diagnosis as part of a science called molecular biology.

Polysaccharides. Carbohydrates made up of long chains of sugar molecules bonded together. Starch and cellulose (found in plants) are two examples.

Porous. Permeable to liquids.

Porphyromonas gingivalis **(PG).** A kind of bacteria found in the mouth and associated with periodontal gum disease. It can evade the immune system and produce enzymes that cause gum inflammation and bone loss. Studies have linked it to cardiovascular disease, rheumatoid arthritis and Alzheimer's disease.

Prebiotic. A group of nutrients that selectively support beneficial bacteria in the mouth, promoting a healthier balance of bacteria for health. Xylitol is an example of an ideal oral prebiotic food. (See also *Probiotic*.)

Prevotella **bacteria.** A group of bacteria that live in low oxygen conditions and are found in the mouth, gut, and female reproductive tract. Some species are associated with periodontal gum disease and systemic infections, whereas others contribute to a healthy digestion by breaking down carbohydrates and proteins in the gut.

Probiotic. Live bacteria or yeasts that may be introduced in supplement form to balance or enhance the natural mix of bacteria found in the gut. These same bacteria may also be found in fermented foods like yogurt, kefir, sauerkraut and kimchi. (See also *Prebiotic*.)

Pterygoid plexus. A network of small veins in an area deep within the face, and with connections to veins near the brain—where blood from the nose, face, and teeth drain into the larger veins of the neck. It is through this pathway that dental infections can sometimes travel to the brain.

Pulp. The soft innermost part of a tooth that contains the tooth's nerves, blood vessels, lymphatic fluids, and cells that can detect and transmit pain sensations to the brain.

Recession (gum). A condition where the gum around teeth moves down the root of the tooth exposing sensitive dentin, an area that can feel sensitive to temperature because it is not shielded by dental enamel.

Recurrent decay. Continued damage to a tooth from decay-forming bacteria in plaque that may attack the edges of an existing filling and even travel around and under the filling.

Remineralization (tooth). The rebuilding of minerals back into enamel to repair and replace missing minerals so that the tooth regains strength.

Retainer. A dental appliance made of plastic or metal and designed to keep teeth in a specific position—often after orthodontic movement. Retainers can be permanently fixed in the mouth or removable, which allows them to be taken out for cleaning.

Root canal. A dental procedure to save a tooth that has suffered damage or infection in the central area. Any damaged or diseased parts are removed, and then a special filling seals the area completely, even to the tips of the roots. This technique requires skill and experience for success, so it is best performed by a specialist called an *endodontist*.

Saliva. A watery liquid produced by salivary glands to keep the mouth healthy, mineralize teeth, fight gum infection, keep the mouth moist, and aid in the processes of digestion, chewing, and swallowing.

Sealant(s). A coating, usually made of plastic, applied to the grooves and crevices in the chewing surfaces of teeth to prohibit entry of bacteria. This concept was developed before the understanding that these areas are an important habitat for beneficial bacteria.

Silica. One of the most abundant naturally occurring minerals on Earth. It is found in sand, glass, ceramics, certain foods, and in certain toothpaste products to support enamel health.

Sorbitol. A sugar alcohol used in many sugar-free foods, which occurs in some fruits but is generally manufactured for commercial use. Sorbitol should not be consumed by children.

Stannous fluoride. One of the least expensive fluoride compounds available and fabricated by a reaction between fluoride and metal. The metal is tin, and it gives stannous fluoride antibacterial effects and an ability to form plugs in the surface of teeth. This is claimed as an advantage, but stannous fluoride can stain teeth and create toxic reactions, thus causing skin sensitivity in the mouth.

Stem cell(s). Unique, undifferentiated cells able to change into many types of specialized cell and renew themselves. They play a crucial role in growth, organ repair, and wound healing.

Streptococcus mutans. A type of mouth bacteria that contributes to plaque formation and tooth decay because it can stick to teeth and produce acids that erode tooth enamel. *S. mutans* can process sugar and carbohydrates but is unable to process xylitol as an energy source.

Sucrose. Most people use this as a table sugar, and it's valued for sweetness. Sucrose is naturally found in fruits and vegetables, including pineapples, peaches, sugar cane, carrots, sweet potatoes, and beets. It is a carbohydrate that can be broken down into glucose and fructose and used by the body for energy or stored.

Sugar alcohol(s). A group of carbohydrates with similar chemical structure. They have less calories than sugar and are commonly used in low calorie or sugar-free foods and drinks.

Sulfide(s)/Sulphide (*British spelling*). A chemical compound that contains sulfur—often in combination with a metal or hydrogen—iron sulfide (*pyrite*), for example (which is called "fool's gold"), and hydrogen sulfide—a gas with the smell of rotten eggs.

Super-saturation. A state when a liquid contains more dissolved particles than normal. This makes the solution unstable and ready to release these extra minerals or particles.

Tartar. Sometimes called calculus and formed when plaque crusts into a hard substance on the outside of teeth. (See also *Plaque.*)

Thorax. The area between the neck and the abdomen housing vital body parts including the heart, lungs, diaphragm and major blood vessels: all protected by the structure of the rib cage.

Thrush. A creamy-white infection of the tongue, cheeks, gums, and tonsils, caused by an overgrowth of *candida albicans*—a yeast that is naturally present in the body in small amounts. The areas can be sore and will bleed if scraped.

Triclosan. A synthetic compound that can kill bacteria and fungi and formerly used in personal care products until it was found to be a hormone disruptor—affecting thyroid and reproductive health, and polluting the soil, water, and environment.

Turmeric. (See *Curcumin.*)

Venous. The blood vessels that carry de-oxygenated blood to the heart, where it is pumped to the lungs and re-oxygenated.

Voussoir arch. An arch created by arranging wedge-shaped stones in a curved design so that downward forces are distributed outwardly and the stones interlock to resist collapse.

White spot lesions. The first stage of a cavity, seen with the naked eye as minerals are lost and the tooth surface weakens and becomes porous.

Xylitol. A health sugar found in trees, fruits, and made by the human body. It has a unique molecular pattern with five carbon atoms (while sugar and sugar alcohols have six). This pentose structure allows xylitol to control plaque's ability to grow and multiply. (See also *Pentose.*)

Zinc. A metallic element that is essential for human health, supporting immune function, growth, and wound healing. It occurs naturally in meat, shellfish, and dairy products.

About the Author

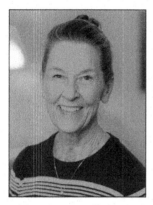

Ellie Phillips, DDS, received her specialty qualifications in pediatric and advanced general dentistry from the University of Rochester, New York. Dr. Phillips is also a graduate of Guy's Hospital Medical School in London and licensed as a dentist in Switzerland. She has worked in many fields of dentistry, including oral surgery, community and general practice, in geriatric, special needs, and cosmetic dentistry. She was faculty and pediatric clinic director at the Eastman Institute for Oral Health in Rochester, NY, where she was worked with professors who were involved in many xylitol studies. Her lifelong interest has been the impact of mouth health on general health and wellness, and this led her to be a founding member of the American Academy for Oral Systemic Health (AAOSH) and a leader in creating a multidisciplinary dental practice at the University of Rochester.

Dr. Phillips has been interviewed extensively by various media outlets and publications both in the US and abroad—including *The Times of London, The New York Times, The New York Post, First for Women, The Daily Mail (UK),* and *FOX News.* She also has an active social media presence that extends to popular apps such as TikTok, Instagram, Facebook, and YouTube, where she has brought her inspiring message of health empowerment to millions of fans and followers throughout the world.

Dr. Phillips lives in Austin, Texas, and continues to share her expertise as a speaker, consultant, and author of articles on topics related to the value and importance of dental health at every stage of life. In addition to being the author of her previous book Mouth Care Comes Clean, Dr. Phillips is the founder of the popular dental health company Zellies.com. Those who wish to learn more about her various experiences with dental excellence and her ongoing efforts to change the world one healthy smile at a time, feel free to visit her website at **https://drellie.com/**.

Index

G

Gum(s)
  disease, 191–192
  pocketing, 56, 168, 185–186
  recession, 187–189

H

Halitosis (bad breath), 26, 94–95, 160, 162, 187
Human Microbiome Project (of 2007), 18, 155
Human Papilloma Virus (HPV), 51–56

I

International Academy of Oral Medicine and Toxicology, 191
Implant(s), 71–72

J

Jawbone(s), 27, 34–36, 68–69, 71–72

L

Listerine, 108–111, 113

M

McKay, Dr. Frederick S., 16, 75
Microbiome. *See* Biome.
Miswak stick, 10, 105
Mouthwash(es), 66, 74, 94, 101, 109, 157

N

National Cancer Institute (NCI), 109
National Health And Nutrition Examination Survey (NHANES), 53, 59
National Institute of Dental Research, 77

O

Oral cancer, 42, 52–54, 65, 81, 183

P

Periodontal disease, 20, 55, 69, 87, 100, 197
Peroxide, 21, 52, 70, 111, 142, 187
Plaque, 37, 46, 63–64, 98–99, 114–115, 143, 168, 186. *See also* Tartar.

R

Rumbelow, Helen (journalist), 63–64, 198

S

Saliva
  acidic, 44–47
  health, 48–51
  stimulated, 57
  sugary, 47–48
Sealant(s)
  toxicity of, 190–191
Semmelweis, Dr. Ignaz, 14–15
Stem cell(s), 21, 27–28, 151, 166, 168–170, 186, 200

T

Tartar. *See* Plaque.
Teeth (baby), 37, 78, 86, 102, 143–146, 179
"Three S" Approach (mouth health), 94–95
Tooth
  extraction, 196
  sensitivity, 139, 142, 187
  whitening, 19–22, 37–39, 96–97, 106–108, 189, 193–194, 201. *See also* Whitening.
Toothbrushing, 12–13, 95–100, 101–108
Turmeric, (See *Curcumin*.)

W

Whitening. *See* Tooth whitening.

X

X-ray(s), 159–161, 180–183, 187–189
Xylitol
  how to use, 127–131
  mints, 89, 124, 131, 146
  pets, not given to, 132

Y

Young children. *See* Children (dental health).

Z

Zellie's, 124–127